WOMEN AND HEART DISEASE: THE REAL STORY

Jacqueline A. Eubany, M.D., FACC, FHRS

LCCN: 2016909583
ISBN: 978-1534909847

Cover design by Michael Ilacqua
www.cyber-theorist.com

Printed in the United States of America

Praise for Women and Heart Disease: The Real Story.

"This is a must read book for all women, especially for those who have family members, or who themselves have risk factors for cardiovascular disease". - Dr Tiffanie Tate-Moore

"This book is a valuable addition to every woman's library." - Dr. Cynthia Cesaire

"Women who are concerned about their health will find this book invaluable" - Dr Fiona Strasserking

"I don't usually read medical books, but when I read the book I learned so much about diabetes. The author did an excellent job explaining things in a language that was very easy to understand. I highly recommend this book" - Andrea Brooks

"As a practicing physician, I recommend this book for my patients, as it explains heart disease in a manner that is easy to understand, and very practical advice to follow." - Dr. Lorraine Thomas

"Highly informative, succinct and to the point. Very well written and is a must read." - Elmer Davis, Three time New York bestselling author.

"Eye opening and comprehensive overview" -Betty Williams

"Dr. Eubany brings awareness of the impact and importance of heart disease, the number one killer of American women, to women's health in a way that is interesting and understandable to everyone." - Dr. Andrew Breiterman

I dedicate this book to my mother, who has inspired me with her courage, strength and insight; and to my nieces, Maya and Hailey, who are just beginning their journey through life, and may God bless them with the same gifts of courage, strength and insight as my mother was given.

ACKNOWLEDGEMENT

I am indebted to my parents, my mother Ollie Eubany, and my father, the late Cosmos Eubany, for all I am today. I am indebted to my mother, for always encouraging me to be the best that I can be, and being extremely supportive of every single endeavor I have ever attempted. I am indebted to my father for teaching me self-discipline and perseverance. I am grateful to all my siblings Lorraine, Bevelyn, Margaret, and Cosmos, plus all my nieces and nephews, for their love, support and encouragement. And lastly I am truly thankful to Andrew for being a solid foundation in my life.

<u>INTRODUCTION</u>

I have always wanted to be a physician for as long as I can remember. I have invariably been drawn to the idea of helping and serving others. I went to medical school wanting to be an obstetrician/gynecologist. My interest in cardiology and more specifically, women and heart disease did not come until much later. Heart disease is very common in my family. I have had many relatives die at young ages from heart disease, and have seen many complications of heart disease related illnesses in my family, from amputation of limbs, to blindness, to being on dialysis. I have witnessed this so frequently, that when I was growing up, I thought that heart disease was an inevitable result of aging. I did not know the contribution of unhealthy lifestyles to heart disease.

As medical school progressed, I became fascinated by the human heart and everything related to it. Then I began to understand how one's action can promote worsening of heart disease. I thought often of a relative of mine who had a stroke and was paralyzed on one side, yet there was no change in her lifestyle habits. I believe the reason for this was her lack of awareness of the linkage between heart disease and poor lifestyle habits.

After finishing medical school, I joined the United States Navy, where I began my training in medicine. In the military I got to travel and live in many different areas in the United States. Living, and working, first as an internal medicine physician, and then later as a cardiologist, I began to notice the disparities in outcomes of heart disease between women and men. I remember an incident when a woman in her 70's was admitted to my service with a diagnosis of gastroenteritis because she came to the emergency room with nausea and vomiting. She was in the ER for many hours, being treated with anti-nausea medications, and it wasn't until she was admitted to my service that we did several tests and discovered she was having a heart attack. She was taken immediately for cardiac catheterization. Her outcome was poor.

Over the years, I found myself getting invitations to speak about heart disease to women in the local community. As I began doing more research on the subject matter, I was shocked at some of the statistics I learned. Although I had experienced some of these disparities in heart disease outcomes between men and women during my short working experience, I didn't realize just how widespread these differences in outcomes were, and I didn't understand why people were not discussing them, and trying to figure out how to bridge these gaps. When I would speak to these small groups of women about heart disease, I was amazed at some of the questions I was asked. I came to realize that many women are not very well educated on heart disease and lifestyle, nor do they realize that heart disease is the number one killer of American women.

Not only does the general public need education on heart disease, but health care providers need education as well. Because women typically don't have the classic symptoms that men have when suffering a heart attack, they get misdiagnosed or diagnosed late in the disease process, leading to poorer outcomes.

The widespread need for women's heart health education inspired me to educate women on heart disease. The purpose of this book is to explain heart disease in a simple manner that is understandable by anyone and everyone, even without a medical background. I attempt to cover frequently asked questions that were asked of me during my small group sessions. I hope you find the information in this book very helpful to you.

"I can do all things through Christ who strengthens me."
Philippians 4:13

Table of Contents

WOMEN & HEART DISEASE: THE REAL STORY.

Angie is a 46-year-old divorced mother of two school-aged children. One morning she was just not feeling her usual self, but wasn't able to articulate what was wrong. Undaunted, the busy mother went about her usual morning routine of getting her children ready and driving them to school, then on to her job. At work, her symptoms worsened. Angie felt hot and sweaty, but attributed that to the peri-menopausal symptoms that were now somewhat familiar. Over the course of the day, she felt a bit nauseated and lightheaded. A couple of times, Angie thought she might pass out so she stopped her work, sat down, and laid her head on the desk until the feeling passed. Angie's coworkers noticed that she looked unusually pale and advised her to go to the doctor's office. Hard working Angie declined, saying there was too much work to be completed that day. As the sole financial provider for her family, the young woman felt she could not afford to take time off. There were too many outstanding bills and her children needed her. Angie hoped she would soon start to feel better.

Her symptoms worsened over the next three to four days. Angie could barely take a couple of steps without having to stop and catch her breath. Desperate to sleep, her bed became a recliner in the living room since she could not breathe when lying flat on her bed. Angie's legs became so swollen she couldn't wear the shoes in her closet. Concern finally forced her to seek medical attention.

Angie went to the emergency room and was admitted to the intensive care unit right away. The attending staff told her that she was suffering from congestive heart failure likely a result of recent changes in her cardiac health, what doctors call a sub-acute heart attack. The time frame of her 'event' was probably several days prior. Because of ignoring symptoms for a few days and her late presentation to the emergency room, the chances that Angie would make a full recovery following aggressive invasive cardiac treatment were low. She had a long and complicated hospital stay. After discharge from the hospital, the busy mother was medically incapacitated and had to go on permanent disability. If Angie had known about her risk for heart attack and had recognized that her symptoms were very serious, she probably would have sought medical attention sooner. In the early intervention scenario, the damage sustained to her heart would not have been so severe.

Heart disease is the leading cause of death in women in the United States (US). According to a published report from the American Heart Association, there are 600,000 deaths annually from heart disease. In 2009, 292,188 women died from heart disease. That number equates to 1 in 3 of *all female deaths*. Heart disease can no longer be thought of as a "man's" disease. Heart disease kills six times as many women as breast cancer! In 2004, 60% more women died from cardiovascular disease than all types of cancer combined.

The ethnic demographics of heart disease vary slightly. In the United States, heart disease is the leading cause of death for both African American and Caucasian women. The deaths from cardiovascular events are considerably higher for African American women than they are for all other ethnic groups, including Caucasian. In 2009, there were 286.1 cardio vascular related deaths per 100,000 African American females compared to 205.7 deaths per 100,000 Caucasian females in the United States. In Hispanic women, heart disease caused roughly the same amount of deaths as cancer that same year. In Native American and Asian American women, heart disease is the second leading cause of death, after cancer.

The rate of death from heart disease for women between the ages of 35 and 54 appears to be on the rise. Despite these numbers, and multiple attempts at education, only 54% of women are aware that heart disease is the number one killer of women in the US. When surveyed, only 53% of women recognized their own symptoms of heart attack enough to call 911. However, about 80% of women would recognize the symptoms of heart attack in other people and call 911 much earlier than they would for themselves.

Stroke is also considered a cardiovascular disease, and is the second leading cause of cardiovascular death in women. In Americans 75 years of age or younger, 55,000 more women die of stroke or cerebrovascular event than men every year. One reason for this distinction is because certain physical conditions are unique to women when compared to their male counterparts. Pregnancy and hormonal therapy place women at a higher risk for blood clots and strokes. Hormonal therapies include oral contraceptives which can be used to treat an assortment of clinical ailments, and hormone replacement therapy which is often prescribed to women in the peri-menopausal and post-menopausal states. Women who take hormone therapy have higher rates of stroke and blood clots than women who do not receive any of these therapies.

Why are women more likely to die from a heart attack than men? Many theories have been proposed over the years. Women generally do not present to emergency rooms with the "classic symptoms" of heart attack that most people are aware of. The familiar picture of this event, which most adults have likely seen, is that of a man grabbing the left side of his chest with his hands, and with an agonizing facial expression that clearly details the severe pain he is experiencing.

Fig 1.

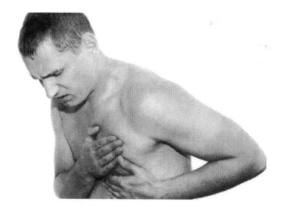

This picture is called the Levine sign, and it has an 80% sensitivity in diagnosing a heart attack. However, women rarely have these well-known signs and symptoms of heart attack. Their "unusual" presentation generally leads to a later diagnosis, and treatment. With late diagnosis, treatment is not as effective in achieving a 100% recovery. Late diagnosis results in higher complication rates and sometimes death. Women's lack of awareness that heart disease is the cause of their symptoms means that they are less likely to seek urgent or emergent medical attention when it is crucial.

Because of her lack of awareness, our patient, Angie, did not seek medical attention immediately. She sought help only after her symptoms had progressed to the point of irreparable heart damage. Like most women, Angie is the sole provider and caretaker of others, and she did not take the time out to take better care of herself. As a result, she ended up on disability, and with an inability to take care of others, let alone herself.

Not all statistics regarding women and heart disease are bleak. The good news is that heart disease and its debilitating effects can be prevented! When heart disease develops despite the implementation of preventative measures, education and awareness can lessen its devastating impact. The purpose of this book is to help women understand heart disease, its symptoms, the risk factors for heart disease and, more importantly, how to prevent this disease from occurring.

"A good heart is better than all the heads in the world."

Edward G. Bulwer-Lytton

NOTES:

WHAT IS HEART DISEASE?

There are several disease states that fall under the heading of heart disease. The one that is familiar to most people is called a myocardial infarction, commonly referred to as a heart attack. Other forms of heart disease include arrhythmias, which are abnormal heart rhythms; stroke, that occurs as a result of blockage to blood vessels of the brain; valvular heart disease, which involves one or more of the heart's four valves; and congestive heart failure, that occurs when the heart fails.

A heart attack happens when one of the blood vessels that supplies the heart with oxygen and nutrients is completely obstructed or blocked, causing a lack of oxygen to the area of the heart that is supplied by that blood vessel. The blockage is usually caused by the accumulation of cholesterol plaque in the artery that grows into the lumen overtime, obstructing it (see fig 2). These cholesterol plaques within the artery can also rupture acutely, causing a cascade of events that lead to blood clot formation, and complete closure of the blood vessel.

Fig 2.

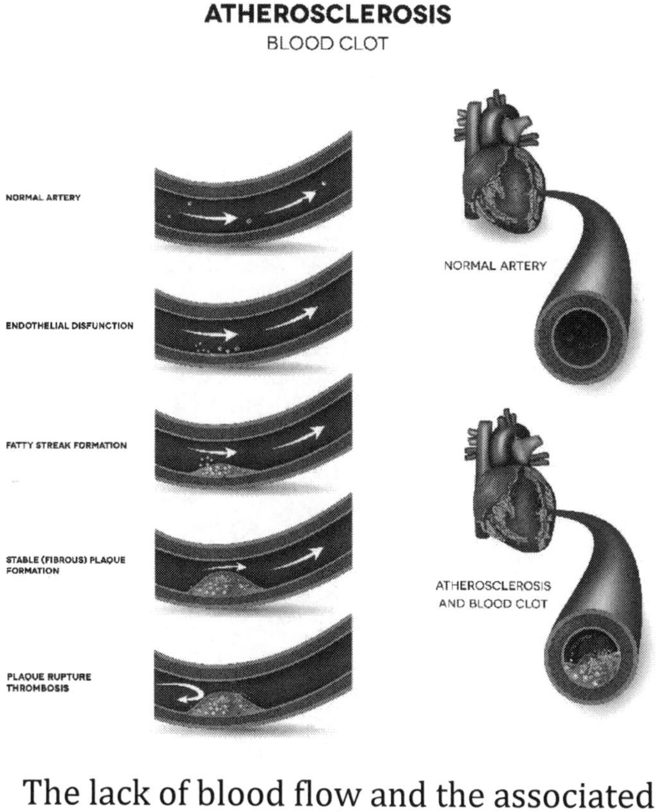

ATHEROSCLEROSIS
BLOOD CLOT

NORMAL ARTERY

ENDOTHELIAL DISFUNCTION

FATTY STREAK FORMATION

STABLE (FIBROUS) PLAQUE FORMATION

PLAQUE RUPTURE THROMBOSIS

NORMAL ARTERY

ATHEROSCLEROSIS AND BLOOD CLOT

The lack of blood flow and the associated lack of oxygen and nutrients to the area of the heart that is supplied by that blocked artery, will lead to heart tissue death. The amount of tissue that dies after an artery is blocked, is dependent on the amount of the heart tissue that is supplied by the blocked artery, and also by the total amount of time that the artery is occluded before medical intervention can reopen it. The more heart tissue death that occurs during an acute occlusion of a coronary artery, and the longer the artery is occluded before any intervention is made to open the blockage, the greater the chance that the heart will not fully recover from this insult. This event will ultimately culminate in heart failure and the inability of the heart to perform its normal function.

The heart's normal function is to contract with a great amount of force to pump oxygen and nutrient filled blood forward to supply all the organs in the body with the energy they need to function normally. In heart failure, either due to heart muscle tissue death from occluded arteries, or from structural damage to the heart muscle contractile apparatus, the heart is unable to pump adequate amounts of blood to other organs in the body. As a result of heart failure, fluid backs up into the lungs and causes congestion in the lungs and liver. People with heart failure experience shortness of breath with the mildest of exertion, and they may have orthopnea – shortness of breath when lying flat – causing them to sleep in a reclined position. People with heart failure may wake up in the middle of the night because of attacks of shortness of breath and coughing which is called paroxysmal nocturnal dyspnea. In heart failure, both legs swell with fluid, and there is an overall weight gain from fluid retention and generalized fatigue with an inability to exercise (see fig. 3). Over time, other body organs do not receive adequate amounts of nutrients or oxygen for energy and begin to fail. The clinical symptoms of *end organ damage* depend on which organ is damaged. For example, if the damage is in the kidney, one would experience decreased urination, increased total body fluid retention, and a buildup of toxins in the body causing lethargy, which could lead to the requirement for dialysis.

Fig 3.

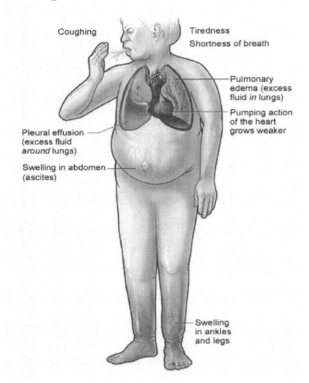

Coughing

Tiredness
Shortness of breath

Pulmonary edema (excess fluid *in* lungs)

Pumping action of the heart grows weaker

Pleural effusion (excess fluid *around* lungs)

Swelling in abdomen (ascites)

Swelling in ankles and legs

Another form of heart disease is called arrhythmia, or an abnormal heart rhythm. Typically, for the heart to contract smoothly and pump an adequate amount of nutrient and oxygen filled blood to the rest of the body, it must generate electrical energy. The electrical impulse begins at the top of the heart and is produced by specialized cells called the *sinus node*, also known as the pacemaker of the heart. This impulse occurs because of the inherent characteristics of these cells at a microscopic level. This impulse is propagated, throughout the heart in a coordinated fashion, and gets translated into mechanical energy that produces a forceful contraction of the heart. Any problem with the generation and propagation of the impulse in a coordinated manner from the top to the bottom of the heart is referred to as an arrhythmia. Arrhythmias are characterized as either being too fast (heart rates above 100 beats per minute), or too slow (heart rates less than 60 beats per minute). Arrhythmias initiated by impulses in the top chambers of the heart, the atria, are referred to as supraventricular arrhythmias. Arrhythmias arising from impulses in the bottom chambers of the heart, the ventricles, are referred to as ventricular arrhythmias. Arrhythmias can be benign, meaning they are of no clinical significance, or they can be malignant, meaning they can lead to sudden cardiac death.

Atrial fibrillation affects 2.7 million people and is one of the most common arrhythmias in the United States. It is triggered by impulses that fire rapidly into the atrium. As a result of its origin in the top chamber of the heart (the atrium), and the rapid impulses that translate into rapid heartbeats, it is called a *supraventricular tachycardia.* In atrial fibrillation, the atrium does not contract in a smooth fashion. Instead, the electrical impulses are rapid and chaotic (see fig. 4). On account of this rapid and ineffective contraction, blood is not adequately emptied from the atrium. Blood lingers in this chamber and can form blood clots. These blood clots can break off and be transported to the brain, causing a stroke. Atrial fibrillation is independently associated with a 4 to 5-fold increased risk of stroke and is responsible for 15-20% of all strokes.

Other examples of abnormal heart rhythms include *complete heart block, sinus node dysfunction,* and *atrial or ventricular tachycardia/fibrillation.*

Fig 4.

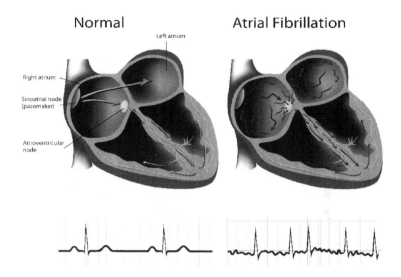

Normal

Atrial Fibrillation

Left atrium

Right atrium

Sinoatrial node
(pacemaker)

Atrioventricular
node

A third form of heart disease is called *valvular heart disease*. The heart has four valves within it, which function as check valves that allow blood to flow in a forward direction. When the valves become damaged for whatever reason, one of two problems may arise. The blood can leak backwards as a result of an incompetent valve, or the valve can become stenotic (which means that its opening is restricted) preventing forward blood flow. Valvular heart disease produces symptoms of chest pain, shortness of breath, and exercise intolerance. It ultimately leads to heart failure if left untreated.

Finally, another form of heart disease is called *congestive heart failure*. Congestive heart failure, as mentioned above, is the inability of the heart to adequately pump oxygen and nutrient-filled blood out of the heart, and to the different organs in the body. Since all the organs in the body need oxygen and require nutrients for energy to function normally, the organs can fail over time. Heart failure can be a primary disorder - that is, a genetic abnormality that leads to inadequate structural development of the heart. Much more commonly, heart failure is the end-stage result of all forms of heart disease.

"A good head and a good heart are always a formidable combination."

Nelson Mandela

NOTES:

RISK ASSESSMENT

Most people develop some form of heart disease in their lifetime, but there are certain risk factors, or behaviors, that place some people at higher risk than others. These risk factors include smoking, physical inactivity, poor diet, obesity, hypertension, diabetes, high cholesterol, and other inheritable diseases like collagen vascular disease. Most of these risk factors can be improved upon by lifestyle modification, but some risk factors, unfortunately, are unalterable, and therefore cannot be changed. Examples of unalterable risk factors include age, ethnicity, and family history.

There are ways to treat and modify one's risk factors to prevent a cardiovascular event from occurring, or to decrease the impact of the disease, if and when it does occur. Modifying your risk factors for cardiovascular disease can decrease your risk of having a heart attack by almost 80%!!!

What are your risks for developing heart disease? (refer to tables 1, 2 and 3).

Classification of cardiovascular risk in women

Table 1

Risk Status	Criteria
High risk (≥ 1 high risk states)	-Clinically manifest heart disease -Clinically manifest cerebrovascular disease -Clinically manifest peripheral arterial disease -Abdominal aortic aneurysm -End stage or chronic kidney disease -Diabetes mellitus -10 yr. Framingham predicted heart disease risk ≥ 10%

Table 2

Risk Status	Criteria
At risk (≥ 1 major risk factors)	-Cigarette smoking -BP > 120/80 or treated hypertension -Total cholesterol > 200mg/dl; HDL-C <50 mg/dl or treated for high cholesterol -Obesity -Poor diet -Physical inactivity -Family history of premature heart disease in first degree relative men < 55 yr. or women < 65yr -Metabolic syndrome -Evidence of advanced subclinical atherosclerosis

At risk **continued** ($\geq$ 1 major risk factors)	-Poor exercise capacity on treadmill test and/or abnormal heart rate recovery after stopping -Collagen vascular disease (lupus, rheumatoid arthritis) -History of gestational diabetes, preeclampsia, pregnancy induced hypertension

Table 3

Risk Status	Criteria
Ideal cardiovascular health	-Total cholesterol < 200mg/dl (untreated)
	-BP < 120/80 mmHg
	-Fasting blood glucose < 100mg/dl (untreated)
	-Body Mass Index < 25kg/m2
	-Abstinence from smoking
	-Physical activity at goal for adults > 20 yr.: $\geq$ 150 min/wk. moderate intensity, $\geq$ 75 min/wk. vigorous intensity, or combination
	-Healthy (DASH-like) diet

"I can't change the direction of the wind, but I can adjust my sails to always reach my destination."

Jimmy Dean

NOTES:

CIGARETTE SMOKING

Beverly is a 43-year-old married mother of a teenage boy who sees her doctor on a routine basis. When Beverly requests a refill on her oral contraceptive medication, she reveals to her provider that she smokes about a pack of cigarettes per day. The middle age woman began smoking in her early twenties, and started by smoking a few cigarettes intermittently but has slowly progressed over the years to smoking a full pack of cigarettes per day. She was diagnosed in the past with borderline high blood pressure, but she says she was never put on medication. It never came up again in subsequent doctor's visits. Her father died when he was 60 years of age from a heart attack. Beverly feels in excellent health and does not believe she has any concerning medical condition.

A couple of years later, Beverly suffered a massive stroke that left her paralyzed on the left side and unable to speak. Unable to breathe on her own, she required a breathing tube. A feeding tube was attached to her stomach because she was unable to swallow any food that was placed in her mouth. Beverly had a long and complicated hospital stay and was finally discharged from the hospital after almost two months.

Cigarette smoking is a major risk factor for cardiovascular disease. The United States Surgeon General calls it "the leading preventable cause of disease and death in the United States." A study showed that of the 2.4 million annual deaths in the US, smoking accounts for 440,000.

According to the American Lung Association, there are roughly 600 ingredients in every cigarette. When a cigarette is lit and burning, these 600 ingredients are converted to more than 7,000 chemicals. A minimum of 69 of these chemicals are known to cause cancer and are extremely poisonous. One of these ingredients, nicotine, is a highly addictive drug. When nicotine is inhaled, it reaches the brain faster than any intravenous drug. Nicotine gives smokers the "buzz" they feel when smoking. It can be as addictive as alcohol, heroin, and cocaine.

Fig. 5.

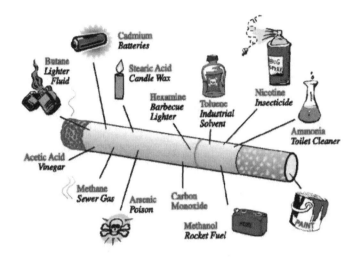

Cigarette smoking is detrimental to most internal organs and causes diseases like cancer, chronic lung disease, heart disease, and blockages in blood vessels throughout the body. In the vascular system, smoking lowers good cholesterol and contributes to cholesterol plaque buildup in the arteries of the heart, increasing a person's risk for heart attack. In the pulmonary system, damage to

40

the lungs decreases one's ability to exercise adequately.

Nicotine is a powerful vasoconstrictor. This means that it causes the blood vessels to contract and contributes to high blood pressure. Other organ systems, which depend on intricate arterial supplies, are damaged by nicotine, including the brain, which may experience strokes; the eyes, leading to cataracts; the kidneys, resulting in kidney failure requiring dialysis; the skin, causing premature wrinkling and hair loss; the arterial system, leading to peripheral vascular disease and lastly, the reproductive system. In women, the reproductive organs are affected by cigarette smoking, and a woman in her reproductive years, who is a smoker, increases her chances of infertility. A discussion of the health effects of tobacco could go on forever, but this is a book about women and heart disease, so we will try to keep the discussion relevant to that topic.

The risk of stroke and cardiovascular events is much higher in women under the age of 50 years who smoke *and* take oral contraceptives. In general, smokers die earlier than nonsmokers. Men who smoke die 13.2 years earlier than men who do not smoke, while women who smoke die 14.5 years earlier than women do not smoke.

Second hand smoke is also dangerous. Second hand smoke is tobacco smoke exhaled by a smoker, and inhaled by a nonsmoker. One study showed that each year, roughly 22,700 to 69,600 uncommonly early deaths are due to second hand smoke. That means, you simply have to be *exposed* to cigarette smoke as a nonsmoker to be impacted negatively. Because of this, the American College of Cardiology recommends that women quit smoking and avoid environmental tobacco smoke. The best way to quit smoking is simply to do it cold turkey. This is a very difficult challenge because the symptoms associated with nicotine withdrawal can be very uncomfortable. Some nicotine withdrawal symptoms include strong cigarette cravings, anxiety, difficulty concentrating, irritability, and the most dreaded of all side effects - increased appetite and weight gain!

There are several options available to help you quit smoking. In terms of pharmaceutical drugs, there are currently seven medications that have been approved by the Food and Drug Administration (FDA) for smoking cessation.

Nicotine-containing medications or nicotine replacement therapies include nicotine patches, nicotine gums, nicotine lozenges, and nicotine sprays or inhalers. Although they contain nicotine, which is addictive, these medications spare users from being exposed to the cancer-causing chemicals found in cigarettes.

The non-nicotine medications that are FDA approved to help quit smoking include bupropion SR (Zyban) and varenicline tartrate (Chantix). When these therapies are used in conjunction with support groups, the success rate of smoking cessation and remaining tobacco free long term is high.

The good news is that quitting smoking does reduce your risk of dying prematurely or from developing chronic disease. The earlier you quit smoking, the more likely you will benefit from a reduced risk of smoking related health issues. Overall, quitting is beneficial for people of all ages.

Smoking has many harmful effects during pregnancy both to mom and baby. Not only does smoking increase the risk of infertility, but when women become pregnant and continue to smoke, the chances for miscarriage, premature birth and/or birth defects are increased. Nicotine exposure can cause the baby's heart to beat rapidly and it slows down breathing movements. Smoking can also cause problems with the placenta. Also known as the afterbirth, the placenta is the organ that connects the unborn baby to the womb. It supplies oxygen and nutrients to the baby, as well as removing the waste products. Smoking reduces the amounts of oxygen and nutrients that are supplied to the baby through the placenta. Smoking can also cause the placenta to separate from the womb, leading to problems like bleeding, premature birth, low birth weight, and even death to the baby and mother. When a smoker's child is born, the baby is at increased risk of chronic lung diseases like asthma. The child is also at increased lifelong risk for allergies, and chronic ear infections. More importantly, the newborn is at increased risk for Sudden Infant Death syndrome (SIDS). SIDS is when an infant dies suddenly and unexpectedly with no obvious cause of death to be found.

Secondhand smoke has the same effect on an unborn baby as firsthand smoke does. Firsthand smoke, of course, is when the mother is the smoker. Quitting smoking at any time during pregnancy is very beneficial to both mom and baby. NOTE that none of the FDA approved medications for smoking cessation are recommended for use during pregnancy. However, if you are a smoker, pregnant, and desire to quit smoking but are having a difficult time, you should talk to your physician about which option is right for you. Nicotine replacement therapy can be an option for you. While this therapy still delivers nicotine to the unborn baby, it limits the infant's exposure to many of the harmful chemicals found in cigarettes, thus decreasing the overall risk to the baby.

For more questions or tips on quitting, please call 1-800-QUIT-NOW. You can also visit the American Heart Association's website (www.heart.org) or that of the American Lung Association (www.lung.org) for additional information.

Some tips that may be helpful to quit smoking:

- Set a quit date.
- Make a list of the benefits of quitting: for example, the benefit to the health of your unborn baby.
- Develop a strong support system, for example, have someone to talk to when the urge to smoke is overwhelming.
- Change habits that promote smoking, such as avoiding people who smoke and places where smoking is allowed, getting rid of cigarettes or lighters around the house, etc.
- Talk to your primary care physician about other options for quitting

"Let my soul smile through my heart and my heart smile through my eyes, that I may scatter rich smiles in sad hearts."
Paramahansa Yogananda

NOTES:

PHYSICAL ACTIVITY

There is a great amount of scientific evidence that supports the fact that physical activity has many health benefits. Exercise is beneficial in healthy individuals, in individuals who are considered to be at risk for disease, and in those with chronic disease. The cardiovascular benefits of physical exercise are extensive and have been widely documented. Exercise lowers blood pressure, reduces bad cholesterol and increases good cholesterol, lowers the risk of type 2 diabetes, lowers the chances of metabolic syndrome, prevents weight gain, and reduces the risk of premature death from cardiovascular disease, along with all other causes of premature death. Physical activity significantly reduces risk factors for cardiovascular disease.

Three kinds of physical activity have been studied in detail to determine their health benefits. These include aerobic exercise, bone strengthening exercises, and muscle strengthening exercises.

AEROBIC EXERCISE:

Aerobic activity, also known as "cardio," is any physical exercise that requires additional effort by the heart and lungs to meet the muscles' increased demand for oxygen. It usually results in increased heart and breathing rates, which in turn raises the heart and lung's efficiency. Aerobic exercise includes activities like cycling, brisk walking, jogging, swimming, vigorous dancing, or any prolonged exercise that requires oxygen during the aerobic energy generating process.

Three components of aerobic activity have been assessed in studies that examined the cardiovascular benefit of exercise. The three components are: intensity, duration, and frequency of aerobic activity. Intensity is divided into two categories: moderate intensity and vigorous intensity aerobic activity. Moderate intensity aerobic activity usually requires a moderate amount of effort usually resulting in a noticeable increase in heart rate. An example of this is brisk walking. Vigorous intensity aerobic activity usually requires greater effort and results in higher heart rates than moderate activity and more rapid breathing. When evaluating these three components of aerobic activity (intensity, duration, and frequency), studies reveal that the most important component in attaining health benefits is the duration of time spent doing aerobic activities. The more time you spend being physically active, the more cardiovascular benefit you achieve. The intensity and frequency of aerobic activity are less significant than the aerobic activity's duration.

Table 4

Moderate intensity aerobic activity	Vigorous intensity aerobic activity
Brisk walking	Running, jogging, hiking uphill
Household chores (scrubbing floors, cleaning, moving light furniture)	Heavy household chores (moving furniture, carrying > 25lbs, walking up and down stairs carrying > 50lbs
Dancing	Swimming laps
Carrying no more than 20 kg	Carrying more than 20 kg
Gardening and yard work (planting, raking, trimming)	Gardening and yard work (shoveling >10lbs, pushing lawn mower)
Water aerobics	Biking fast more than 10 mph
Sports (golf, Frisbee, badminton)	Competitive sports (football, basketball, soccer, lacrosse)

The intensity of aerobic activity varies from person to person and is dependent on a person's physical fitness level and overall health. How do you know whether you are exercising moderately or vigorously? If you can talk but cannot sing the words to a song while exercising, then you are more than likely participating in a moderate intensity workout. If you can barely say more than one or two words before pausing to catch your breath, then you are likely doing an activity of vigorous intensity.

Muscle strengthening exercises:

Muscle strengthening exercises are activities that strengthen muscle by either lifting heavy objects or using resistance like the body's weight or elastic bands. Cardiovascular benefits have been shown to occur with this form of exercise just as with aerobic activity. The cardiovascular benefits seen with muscle strengthening exercise are more dependent on the amount of time spent doing this activity than the frequency or intensity of the exercise.

Bone strengthening exercises:

Bone strengthening exercises are a combination of low impact aerobic activity and muscle strengthening activity that is designed to build and maintain bone density. This form of physical activity has no proven cardiovascular benefit, but it does benefit other chronic medical conditions. As people age, they lose bone mineral. When too much bone mineral is lost, they become osteopenic. As more mineral is lost, osteoporosis develops. When osteoporosis sets in, the bones become thin and brittle and can break more easily with minor trauma like falls. Bone strengthening exercise helps prevent the loss of bone mineral that occurs with aging. It also helps patients avoid any associated debilitating fractures that could prevent the aerobic and muscle strengthening exercise which is so important to cardiac health. Any weight bearing activity is good for bone strengthening, including walking, tai-chi, or Pilates.

Duration and intensity:

What level of activity do you need to attain the desired cardiovascular benefits? According to the guidelines published in the *Journal of the American College of Cardiology*, 'women should engage in a minimum of 150 minutes a week of moderate aerobic activity, 75 minutes a week of vigorous aerobic activity, or some combination of moderate and vigorous activity'. Aerobic activity should be performed in episodes of at least 10 minutes and should preferably be spread throughout the week. For additional cardiovascular benefits, moderate aerobic activity should be increased to 300 minutes (5 hours) per week and vigorous aerobic activity to 150 minutes (2.5 hours) per week, or to an equivalent combination of both. In general, two minutes of moderate activity are equivalent to one minute of vigorous activity, so you can adjust your exercise time accordingly.

The guidelines for muscle strengthening exercises are vague. There is no mention about any specific duration or intensity for this kind of exercise. The general recommendation is to perform muscle-strengthening activities that involve all major muscle groups on two or more days per week. These major muscle groups include the legs, back, hips, shoulder, chest, abdomen, and arms. When working each muscle group, you want to continue until each muscle group fatigues to the point that you need help to complete the activity. Only then do you gain health benefits from muscle strengthening exercises. This type of fatigue is produced by 8-12 repetitions of one movement, 1 set. As you get stronger, you can increase to 2-3 sets for each muscle group. You can perform muscle-strengthening exercises on the same day you do your aerobic exercise. Or you can do them on separate days; the key is to do them! Remember that you cannot substitute the amount of time you spend doing muscle-strengthening exercise for aerobic activity. For cardiovascular health benefit, you need to do 150-300 minutes of aerobic activity regardless of how much time you spend doing muscle strengthening exercises.

Women who are not able to perform moderate physical activity for 150 minutes per week should start at whatever level they can and gradually increase over weeks to months until they reach the recommended amount of exercise. Any amount of exercise is always better than no exercise at all. Overall, two and a half hours a week of exercise is a reasonable and an achievable goal. To put it into perspective, this is roughly the same amount of time you would spend watching your favorite movie.

Women who are physically active and already meet the minimum guidelines of 150 minutes per week are encouraged to try to increase their exercise time up to 300 minutes a week. Highly active people can and should maintain their current activity level. Pregnant and postpartum women also benefit from regular exercise and can follow the same guidelines. There is strong evidence that moderate intensity exercise during pregnancy is not detrimental to the fetus. As a matter of fact, there is some evidence - although not conclusive - that suggests moderate exercise may even reduce pregnancy complications.

It is not unusual to be hesitant about starting an exercise regimen for fear of getting injured or having a heart attack. However, cardiovascular events during physical activity are rare. The risk is higher when an inactive person suddenly decides to take part in extremely vigorous activity. If you want to begin an exercise program and you have chronic medical problems, I advise you to see your physician. Have them give you recommendations for the best exercise program to fit your current fitness level. Once you have figured out what your starting level of physical activity should be, you can slowly and confidently increase the duration and intensity of exercise to build up your fitness level. Overall, the benefits of physical activity are much greater than those of physical inactivity.

There are many ways that these physical activity guidelines can be integrated into your daily schedule. I will offer examples of three fictitious characters with different levels of physical activity and explain how the goals put forth by these guidelines can be achieved.

Cindy is a physically inactive person. She has never been interested in regular exercise. Her doctor knows she needs to start and Cindy agrees that it is never too late to take charge of her health and longevity. To implement the guidelines and increase her activity level, she can begin by walking for 10 minutes a day for

3 days out of the week. By week 4, she can add an additional 5 minutes to her walk and increase the time by 5 more minutes every 2 weeks. If she keeps at this pace, by the 11th week she will be walking 30 minutes a day 3 days a week, giving her a total of 90 minutes of moderate physical activity each week. By the 12th week, Cindy can look for other activities that involve moderate-intensity physical activity that she can perform on the weekend. Signing up for a scheduled class or event increases the likelihood that Cindy will participate. Examples of this might be taking a dance aerobics class, swimming or biking with a friend, or ballroom dancing. She can do one of these activities for 1 additional hour a week, bringing her total time up to 150 minutes a week. She can then add 10 minutes of muscle strengthening exercise 2 nights a week using hand weights indoors while watching television, outdoors while watching the sunset or at the gym. In about 3 to 4 months, she will reach the minimum guidelines for physical activity where cardiovascular benefits are attained. Once she becomes comfortable with this routine, Cindy can continue to increase the amount of time she spends doing moderate

activity at whatever rate she feels is comfortable, until she reaches the next level of fitness. Taking this process one step at a time will help the inactive person be successful in reaching the recommended levels of heart healthy exercise.

Darlene considers herself to be pretty physically active. She attends spinning class at her local gym two days a week for an hour each time. She would like to increase her physical activity to meet the guidelines for cardiovascular fitness. She can do this by adding another spin class or aerobics class to her weekly schedule. Over time, she can add 2 days of a 60-minute brisk walking. She can then increase the intensity of the brisk walk to jogging. One minute of jogging is roughly equivalent to two minutes of brisk walking. Over the course of two or three months, she would have increased her moderate physical activity to 300 minutes per week. This activity, along with muscle strengthening activities two other days a week should get her to her goal.

Edna is a 75-year-old woman who had a hospital admission for chest pain. After her workup was completed, she learned that she had a small heart attack and was diagnosed with atrial fibrillation. She was "tuned up" and given a pacemaker to prevent her heart rate from getting too low in the future. Edna was initially terrified that any strenuous activity would give her another heart attack and kill her. Her doctor reassured Edna that exercise is beneficial to her rehabilitation and in the prevention of additional heart attacks. Edna then enrolled in a cardiac rehabilitation program where she underwent supervised physical activity, until she no longer needed supervision. The renewed and enthusiastic 75-year-old continued her physical activity by first increasing the number of days, spent doing physical activity. Then she increased the duration of her physical activity until she reached her goal.

Following a heart attack, it is commonplace to take part in a cardiac rehabilitation program, with supervised instruction in exercise. With training and success, a patient will graduate to unsupervised physical activity. For any elderly inactive person, vigorous aerobic activities should be avoided initially to reduce the risk of injury. One should begin with stretching exercises prior to moderate physical activity. Moderate physical activity should be performed for up to 10 minutes a day and increased gradually, by first increasing the number of days of activity and then increasing the amount of time spent doing the activity. Classes and instruction in stretching and exercise are available at gyms, community centers, and other community sources. If the elderly person also has chronic medical problems, he or she should talk with a doctor about developing a physical activity plan that is achievable. In almost all situations, a tailored exercise program can be created.

The guideline recommendations for physical activity in a patient who needs to lose weight or maintain weight loss are somewhat different. In addition to a reduced caloric intake, a minimum of 60 - 90 minutes of moderate physical activity on most days, and preferably all days of the week are advised. If the person is able to do vigorous physical activity without hurting themselves, that is ultimately better when done correctly. Body weight does not determine the health benefits received from exercising, so maintaining the minimal level of physical activity that has cardiovascular benefits will be advantageous no matter how much your weight fluctuates.

"It does not matter how slowly you go as long as you do not stop."
Confucius

NOTES:

DIET

A healthy diet is just as important as any other preventative measure taken to improve heart health. The goals of a heart healthy diet are to lower your body's total cholesterol level. Along with lowering the body's total cholesterol, a heart healthy diet should also aim to reduce the body's bad cholesterol, known as low-density lipoprotein (LDL), and to increase the body's good cholesterol, the high-density lipoprotein (HDL) cholesterol. A heart healthy diet has been scientifically proven to be beneficial. It lowers cholesterol and blood pressure while keeping weight under control, which therefore lowers the overall risk of having a cardiovascular event. You may be eating ample and appropriate quantities of food, but if the food that you feed your body does not have the nutrients needed for it to stay healthy, there is little benefit to those calories. Listed below are the American Heart Association's dietary recommendations for a heart healthy diet.

Heart healthy diet recommendations:

- Consume a diet that is rich in fruits and vegetables. The fruits and vegetables rich with micronutrients tend to be the ones with deep color like dark green, deep orange, and yellow. Good examples are fruits and vegetables like carrots, peaches, and spinach.

- Choose whole grains and high-fiber foods like brown rice and quinoa.

- Eat oily fish that contain omega-3-fatty acids at least twice a week (8 ounces per week). Examples of these oily fish include salmon, mackerel, herring, and sardines. Omega-3-fatty acids are also available in pill form and may be considered therapy in women with high cholesterol for primary and secondary prevention of cardiovascular events. In other words, it can prevent a first heart attack in people who have never had a heart attack. And it can prevent a second heart attack in those who *have* had a heart attack. The recommended dose is 1800 mg per day.

- Decrease your intake of saturated fats to no more than 5-6% of your total calories. Replace these fats with polyunsaturated or monounsaturated fats like olive oil or canola oil.

- Cut trans-fats back to less than 1% of your total caloric intake. Trans-fats increase blood levels of bad cholesterol (LDL), and lower blood levels of good cholesterol (HDL). They are usually found in processed foods made with hydrogenated vegetable oils.

- Limit your cholesterol intake to less than 300 mg per day by avoiding egg yolks and whole fat dairy products and selecting lean meats and meat alternatives like beans and tofu, as well as nonfat and low-fat dairy products.

- Decrease your daily sodium intake to less than 2300 mg per day (a teaspoon of salt), or fewer than 1500 mg (less than ¾ teaspoons of salt) if you have high blood pressure, diabetes, or chronic kidney problems. Avoid processed foods that contain high amounts of sodium. Of note, a 1500-mg daily intake of salt does not apply to those who sweat a lot and therefore lose large amounts of salt in their sweat, such as competitive athletes or those whose jobs require moderate to heavy physical activity.

- Consume alcohol in moderation. For women, this is defined as one drink a day.

- Avoid food and drinks with added sugar, like fructose, glucose, and corn syrup. Women should consume no more than 100 calories or 6 teaspoons of added sugar daily.

- Pregnant or breastfeeding women should avoid fish that are high in mercury, including swordfish, shark, and mackerel.

There are different diet plans that have been studied and proven to have cardiovascular benefits. I am going to talk briefly about four of them: The Mediterranean diet, the DASH diet, the TLC diet, and low carbohydrate diets.

The Mediterranean diet is a healthy eating plan based on Mediterranean-style cooking. This diet is rich in fiber, nutrients, polyunsaturated fatty acids like omega-3-fatty acids, and antioxidants. It incorporates plenty of fruits, vegetables, whole grains, and olive oil. It limits the amount of red meats consumed, favoring fish and poultry instead. This diet also incorporates a moderate amount of wine consumption, specifically red wine, with no more than five ounces of wine for women daily. Research shows that this diet plan prevents heart disease, reduces the risk of a second heart attack and death from a heart attack, and increases the efficiency of cholesterol-lowering drugs like statins. Premenopausal women who choose to begin this diet should eat foods rich in iron and vitamins. In addition, since there is very limited consumption of dairy products in this diet plan, women should consult their doctors about possibly taking a calcium supplement. For more information on the Mediterranean diet, please visit the website, www.mayoclinic.org.

Fig 6.

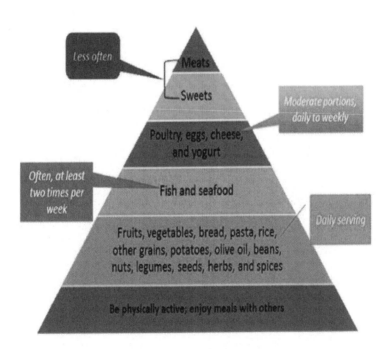

The Dietary Approaches to Stop Hypertension (DASH) diet is a salt restrictive diet that has been shown to help lower blood pressure and decrease the risk of stroke, diabetes, and heart failure. The initial DASH diet was not intended for weight loss, but there have since been modifications that include a weight loss plan and a vegetarian plan. The plan advocates for eating more fresh fruits and vegetables every day, modest amounts of protein (no more than 18% of the total day's calories), whole grains, nuts, legumes, monounsaturated fatty acids like olive oil, and a low sodium intake. The general recommendation is to decrease the amount of sodium in the diet to 2300 mg or less per day. This diet is also rich in nutrients like potassium, magnesium, and calcium and is high in fiber. It is recommended that patients take in at least 30 grams of fiber per day. Other goals include limiting your daily carbohydrate and cholesterol intake. For more on the DASH diet, visit their website at www.dashdiet.org.

Fig. 7.

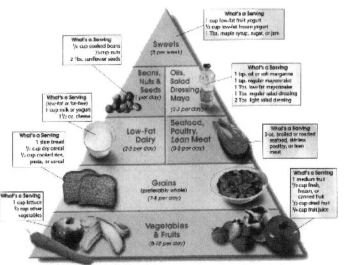

The Therapeutic Lifestyle Changes (TLC) diet, was created by the National Institute of Health's National Cholesterol Education Program, as a heart healthy diet. It has been shown to lower bad cholesterol (LDL cholesterol) and increase good cholesterol (HDL cholesterol), decreasing the risk of a cardiovascular event. There are three main foundations of the TLC diet:

- Changes in diet, including
  o Decreasing daily amounts of saturated fats (less than 7% of the total caloric intake), trans-fat, and cholesterol (<200 mg of daily cholesterol).
  o Increasing the amounts of monounsaturated fats like olive oil and canola oil.
  o Increasing the amounts of soluble fiber.
  o Limiting sodium intake to less than 2400 mg daily.
  o Weight loss and maintenance: For females with a waist circumference greater than 35 inches, the recommendation is to lose weight to decrease cardiovascular risk (more on waist circumference and cardiovascular risk in a later section).
  o Daily physical activity for at least 30 minutes every day.

Low carbohydrate diet. There are many different types of low carbohydrate diets out there. These diets limit carbohydrate intake, but place no restrictions on protein intake. There is a lot of discussion about whether or not these low carbohydrate diets increase a person's risk for cardiovascular disease, as they tend to promote the ingestion of saturated fats and heavy amounts of protein. These are generally not considered heart healthy meal options. Studies do show that low carbohydrate diets lower triglyceride levels (the main fat-carrying particle in the blood) and increase HDL (good cholesterol). However, the general recommendation is that if you do decide to go on a moderately low carbohydrate diet, you should choose protein and fat options that are heart healthy. Examples of heart healthy protein and fat include lean proteins like fish and poultry; and polyunsaturated fats like olive oil and canola oil. Recently published studies indicate a 30% reduction in the risk of heart disease in women and a 20% reduction in the risk for type 2 diabetes in women who opt for low carbohydrate diets high in vegetable sources of protein and fat.

"Man has made many machines, complex and cunning, but which of them indeed rivals the workings of his heart?"
Pablo Casals

NOTES:

ALCOHOL

Alcohol, in moderate doses, may have some cardiovascular benefits. For women, moderation is defined as one drink a day. This can include 12 ounces of beer or a wine cooler, 5 ounces of wine, 1.5 ounces of 80-proof liquor, or 1 ounce of 100-proof spirits. The heart benefits that are associated with alcohol consumption include raising the good cholesterol (HDL). High levels of HDL are protective against the development of atherosclerosis, or cholesterol plaque buildup in arteries. Another beneficial effect of moderate alcohol consumption is its antioxidant effects. Antioxidants help remove dangerous particles that form as byproducts when food gets converted to energy. These dangerous particles, called free oxygen radicals, cause damage to organs and systems. A third beneficial effect of moderate alcohol consumption has to do with its effects on blood clots. Alcohol has been shown in studies to reduce the risk of blood clot formation via a substance contained within it called resveratrol which is found in many plants and plant products such as grape skins. A reduction in the ability to form clots may reduce the rates of heart attacks and strokes.

Research suggests that the health benefits of alcohol are greater with wine consumption, more specifically, red wine, than any other form of alcohol in the marketplace. Red wines contain flavonoids and other antioxidants which have a protective effect on the blood vessels and the heart. The body produces substances called *free oxygen radicals*, which can cause damage to different organs and systems. Flavonoids and other antioxidants contained in red wine act to stabilize the free oxygen radicals to prevent them from causing destruction to organs and systems in the body.

Wine is the only alcoholic product with strongest evidence showing a direct connection between drinking it in moderation and an increase in good cholesterol or HDL levels. This link between moderate alcohol consumption and cardiovascular benefit is still not 100% established, as it remains unclear whether the benefits reported from the studies were from the alcohol itself or the healthy lifestyle habits also adopted by the individuals enrolled in the trial. These healthy lifestyle habits include increased physical activity and a heart healthy diet. As a result, the American Heart Association recommends that those who do not already drink should NOT start drinking just to reap these benefits, as similar benefits can be obtained in other ways, such as increasing physical activity and following a heart healthy diet. If you do drink, do so in moderation, as outlined above.

Fig. 8.

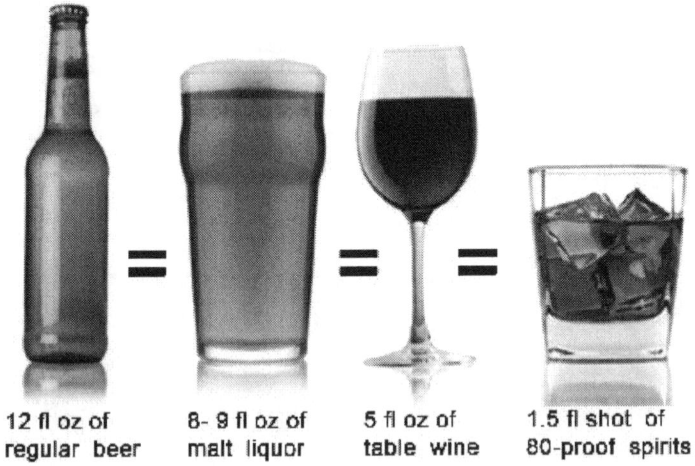

| 12 fl oz of regular beer | 8- 9 fl oz of malt liquor | 5 fl oz of table wine | 1.5 fl shot of 80-proof spirits |

Consuming more than moderate amounts of alcohol is harmful. It can result in high blood pressure, high cholesterol, obesity, stroke, cardiac arrhythmias, heart failure, and sudden cardiac death. Women who are pregnant should not consume any form of alcohol.

"Our greatest weakness lies in giving up. The most certain way to succeed is always to try just one more time."

Thomas A. Edison

NOTES:

HEALTHY WEIGHT

What is a healthy weight? The most popular tool used to calculate healthy weight is the Body Mass Index (BMI). BMI looks at whether your weight is healthy for your height. Research shows that BMI correlates with direct measurements of body fat. You can compute your BMI by multiplying your weight in pounds by 703 and then dividing this number by your height in inches squared. If this sounds too complicated, you can visit the website http://bmicalculator.cc/ and enter in your weight and height, and your BMI will be calculated for you.

A BMI less than 18.5 is considered underweight, and a BMI of 30 and above is considered obese. If your BMI is from 18.5–24.9, you are at a normal weight, while 25–29.9 is considered overweight. A recent study published in the *New England Journal of Medicine* showed a strong correlation between BMI and mortality or death rates. A BMI score of less than 18.5 (underweight) and >25 (overweight and obese) were associated with higher death rates. The lowest mortality rate was seen for a BMI from 22.5–24.9.

Although there is a strong correlation between BMI, and the risk of developing disease and death, one must also remember that BMI is only one factor in the grand scheme of things. Other aspects need to be taken into account when determining a person's risk of developing disease or risk of death from a cardiovascular event. Along with factors mentioned in different parts of this book (such as physical inactivity and high blood pressure), abdominal fat, or waist circumference is also an important risk factor for developing heart disease.

Abdominal or visceral fat has been shown in studies to be more detrimental to health than any other area of the body where fat accumulates, like the thighs and hips. Abdominal fat is associated with an increased risk for heart disease and diabetes. According to a study by the National Institute of Health, a waist size greater than 35 inches in women should be a cause for concern as it correlates with an increase in cardiovascular risk. Another study revealed that women with waist sizes greater than 35 inches had double the risk of death from heart disease than women with waist size less than 28 inches. This risk increased with each additional inch gained and was independent of the person's BMI. In other words, the BMI did not matter as much as waist size in this study. An elevated risk of cardiovascular events was observed even in those whose BMI was considered normal, if they had an abdominal circumference of greater than 35 inches.

Measuring your waist size can be an easier way to keep track of your cardiovascular risk. If you notice an increasing circumference; you can increase your physical activity or decrease your caloric intake to get your abdominal circumference back under 35 inches. To measure your waist circumference, use a measuring tape around your waist at the level of your navel.

Fig. 9.

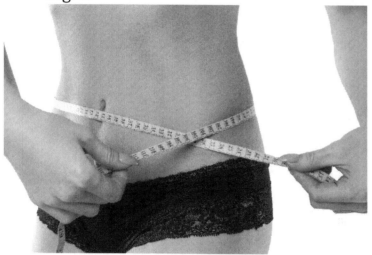

There are many other ways to measure body fat, including underwater weighing, which uses water to determine the body fat to lean mass ratio, dual-energy x-ray absorptiometry (DXA), that measures how much an x-ray dissipates in tissue, skinfold thickness measurements that uses calipers to pinch skin and measures the quantity pinched, and isotope dilutions, a complex and detailed assessment of body composition. These more technical and precise methods are complex, and may yield results that are not intermethod comparable, and will likely require trained personnel to assist in their calculation. These methods can also be quite expensive. Measuring your waist circumference using a simple tape measure is easier to do, free, reproducible, and can provide the same risk assessment.

"Knowing is not enough; we must apply. Willing is not enough, we must do."

Johann Wolfgang Von Goethe

NOTES:

WEIGHT LOSS AND MAINTENANCE

Weight loss, and maintaining that healthy weight, has been shown to lower the risk of heart disease, stroke, diabetes, and high blood pressure. Weight loss and maintenance can be quite difficult because they usually require the implementation of permanent lifestyle changes which include healthy diet choices and an increase in physical activity.

In addition to a poor diet and physical inactivity, other factors that contribute to weight gain include genetics and sleep deprivation. A lack of sleep has been shown to contribute to weight gain likely due to the associated decrease in physical activity, as tired people tend not to exercise. Sleep deprivation can also contribute to weight gain by causing an increase in caloric intake. For example, if you are sleep deprived, you lack the energy required to do your job at work, so you may end up snacking on high calorie foods like donuts and cookies to keep your energy level up. A lack of sleep slows down your metabolism and also produces an imbalance in the hormones that regulate appetite.

There are two hormones that control appetite. They are known as ghrelin and leptin. Ghrelin is the hormone that tells you when to eat, and leptin signals you to stop eating. When you are sleep deprived, you have more of the ghrelin hormone, which causes you to eat more, and less leptin, leaving you with an inability to know when to stop eating.

People with chronic medical problems like diabetes can have an especially difficult time with weight loss. Patients who cannot lose weight in a conventional fashion and whose weight is contributing to the worsening of chronic medical problems might consider weight loss medications or some form of surgical alternative. I strongly recommend consulting your physician if you have chronic medical problems, are overweight and are having difficulty losing weight in the conventional fashion. After listening to all the options offered by your health care provider, you can then make an informed decision about medication versus surgical options for weight loss.

"There is only one corner of the universe you can be certain of improving, and that's your own self."

Aldous Huxley

NOTES:

HYPERTENSION

Francie is a 56-year-old female who sees the doctor for a follow up visit for high blood pressure. During her last two visits, Francie's blood pressure was noted to be elevated. On this visit, her blood pressure is also elevated. She is given the diagnosis of hypertension. Francie is taken aback by this diagnosis! She is shocked because she has never felt any symptoms and doesn't understand why she needs treatment for this. Francie has no chronic medical problems, but is slightly overweight. She reports being under a great deal of stress at work, and with family responsibilities. She doesn't get much sleep at night, and she estimates that she sleeps four to five hours every night. Francie doesn't do any regularly scheduled exercises, she has no fitness regimen, and she is not a smoker, but she loves to drink a glass or two of wine after a long and hard day. She wants to understand the reason for this diagnosis and learn what she can do about it other than taking medications.

Hypertension is a serious condition that affects one in three adults in the United States. Before age 50, women have a lower incidence of hypertension than men. After reaching 55 years of age, the incidence is similar in men and women, and as women age even more the incidence of hypertension exceeds that seen in men. By age 70, there is an 80–90% incidence of hypertension in women.

High blood pressure, also known as hypertension, occurs when blood is pumping with too much force against the artery. Normal, healthy arteries are usually smooth and stretchy, allowing the blood to flow through with ease. Over time, the blood vessels develop scar tissue build up or cholesterol plaques that cause them to narrow and become stiff. This results in blood pumping with a great deal of force to get the same amount of blood flowing to all the organs of the body.

Blood pressure readings consist of two measurements: the systolic pressure (the top number) and the diastolic pressure (the bottom number). The systolic pressure represents the pressure generated when the heart beats and pumps blood out of the heart and into the arteries; this is usually the maximum pressure. The diastolic pressure represents the pressure in the blood vessel when the heart relaxes after it pumps. This is usually the minimum pressure.

The blood pressure guidelines are as follows:

Table 5

Definition	Systolic (mmHg)	Diastolic (mmHg)
Normal	Less than 120	Less than 80
Prehypertension	120–139	80–89
Stage 1 hypertension	140–159	90–99
Stage 2 hypertension	160 or above	100 or above

As a side note, patients with diabetes or chronic kidney disease are considered to have high blood pressure when their BP readings are greater than 130/80 mmHg.

Causes of hypertension:

There are two main categories of high blood pressure: primary hypertension and secondary hypertension. Primary hypertension accounts for about 90-95% of elevated blood pressure, and its cause is not clear. Secondary hypertension makes up 5-10% of all high blood pressure cases, and is usually a result of other medical problems that a person might have.

Causes of secondary hypertension include the following:

• **Hormonal disorders**: There are two main organs or glands in the body that produce hormones whose levels can affect blood pressure. These two glands are the adrenal glands and the thyroid gland. The adrenal glands are small glands that sit on top of each kidney. The adrenal glands produce a variety of hormones, including adrenalin and steroids, which cause a variety of effects on multiple organ systems of the body. Overproduction of the steroid hormones called cortisol and aldosterone will result in high blood pressure. The thyroid gland is located at the base of the neck, just below the Adam's apple, about where a bowtie would sit on the neck. The thyroid gland produces hormones that regulate growth and the rate of function of many organ systems in the body. Too much thyroid hormone production, called hyperthyroidism, or too little thyroid hormone production, termed hypothyroidism, can lead to high blood pressure.

- **Obesity:** This condition has been linked to elevated blood pressure. Obesity is associated with an increase in blood flow, dilation of blood vessels and an increase in the total amount of blood that the body pumps. This then causes an alteration in certain organs involved in maintaining the balance between pressure in blood vessels and overall blood volume leading to hypertension.

- **Kidney disorders:** This is the most common cause of secondary hypertension. There are many kidney disorders that result in hypertension. A thorough discussion of all the kidney abnormalities that cause hypertension is complicated and beyond the scope of this book.

- **Sleep apnea:** A link between sleep apnea and high blood pressure has been made in recent years. Sleep apnea occurs when people stop breathing for short periods of time at night, which often manifests as snoring. These periods with inadequate amounts of oxygen lead to damage to the blood vessels and an ineffective means of regulating blood pressure. Sleep apnea has also been linked with cardiac rhythm problems.

- **Abnormalities of cardiac anatomy:** The aorta is a large artery in the body that is connected to the heart. It receives all the blood that is pumped out of the heart, as well as the pressure that is transferred from the force of contraction of the heart. This large vessel is usually very pliable and can accept the high pressures and volume coming into it from the heart. There is a genetic abnormality called coarctation of the aorta, where a small segment of the aorta is narrow and stiff. With this narrow and stiff segment, the pressure from the force of contraction does not easily get absorbed by the artery and it results in hypertension. The treatment of this disorder requires surgical intervention.

• **Pregnancy:** In the US, 6-8% of pregnancies are complicated by high blood pressure. Hypertension during pregnancy can be potentially life threatening for both the mother and the baby. High risk pregnant patients should be closely monitored by a physician.

• **Drugs:** Many prescription medications, over-the-counter drugs, and herbal supplements, can cause or worsen high blood pressure. Some examples include oral contraceptive pills, hormone replacement therapy, antidepressants, pain relievers, etc. If you have hypertension and are being treated with medications for it, be sure to make your physician aware of any and all prescription, over-the-counter, and/or herbal medications that you are taking. As these medications can interfere with medical treatment of your hypertension.

- **Diabetes:** 60-80% of people with diabetes will develop hypertension. Diabetes causes hypertension by contributing to stiffening of the blood vessels. It speeds up the process of cholesterol and fatty buildup in vessels. Because of this effect of diabetes on blood vessels, the definition of hypertension in diabetic patients is different than in patients without diabetes. Hypertension in diabetic patients is defined as greater than 130/80 mmHg, whereas in nondiabetic patients, it is defined as greater than 140/90 mmHg.

Diagnosis of hypertension:

The American Heart Association recommends that at least three blood pressure measurements taken on at least two different visits to the primary care office be elevated before a diagnosis of hypertension is made. To check a patient's blood pressure, a cuff is placed around the upper arm. The cuff has a gauge on it called a sphygmomanometer, where the blood pressure numbers are displayed. The cuff is inflated slowly, squeezing the arm until the health care provider does not hear a heart sound with the stethoscope. The air is then let out slowly, and the number noted on the dial with the first audible heart sound is the systolic blood pressure. The cuff continues to be deflated until the last heart sound is heard. The number noted on the dial when the last sound is heard is the diastolic blood pressure.

You can also use an ambulatory blood pressure monitor, or a home blood pressure monitoring kit to monitor blood pressures on more regular bases. However, home blood pressure monitoring kits can give erroneous values. I would recommend taking your home kit to your physician's office and comparing its readings to the office machine's readings which are calibrated and accurate, before using your machine at home. If you do have high blood pressure, please seek advice from your physician about how often to check and record your BP at home. This data will assist in your treatment. If your blood pressure is above 180/110 mmHg, you should seek emergency treatment.

Lifestyle modification measures to lower high blood pressure:

Modifying some risk factors for hypertension are out of your control. For example, you cannot change your age, ethnicity, or family history. However, not all risk factors are beyond your control. There are some healthy lifestyle habits that can be adopted to decrease your risk for developing hypertension. These healthy lifestyle habits may be as effective as taking a single blood pressure medication, and can delay the need for medication therapy for hypertension.

Here is a list of some of the lifestyle changes that can help lower high blood pressure:

- Increase physical activity (at least 30 mins/day most days of week). Studies have shown that people who are physically active have a 20–50% lower risk of developing hypertension than those who are not.
- Moderate alcohol use (12 ounces of beer or a wine cooler, 5 ounces of wine, 1.5 ounces of 80-proof liquor daily), if you do drink alcohol. If you don't drink, the recommendation is not to begin.
- Reduce your dietary salt intake (no more than 1500 mg per day).
- Maintain a normal, healthy weight (BMI: 20–25 kg/m^2).
- Eat a healthy diet. The DASH diet, which was discussed in greater detail in a previous section of this book, has been

shown to be effective in lowering blood pressure. A low sodium or vegetarian diet are also effective in reducing blood pressure. Other nutrients that may be beneficial include garlic, omega-3-fatty acids, and high-calcium and high-potassium diets.

- Reduce stress and anxiety levels and get plenty of sleep (7–9 hrs.).
- Regularly monitor your blood pressure at home.
- Reduce your caffeine intake.

Alternative approaches to treating hypertension have also been getting a lot of press. Some of these include herbal therapies like snakeroot, tetrandrine, ginseng, and hawthorn. Nutritional supplements, including coenzyme Q10, omega-3-fatty acids, and amino acids, as well as biofeedback and relaxation techniques like meditation and acupuncture, have been touted as useful approaches also. The safety and efficacy of herbal therapies have not been thoroughly studied, so it is important to talk to your doctor if you are taking these medications or if you plan to, especially if you are already taking prescription medications for chronic medical problems.

Acupuncture has been studied as a means of lowering blood pressure. Results have been mixed, with some controversies on how the studies were performed. More research needs to be done to determine if it is in fact efficacious.

Meditation:

Several risk factors for heart disease have been mentioned, but one risk factor that is seldom discussed is stress and its effect on heart disease. When under stress, your body produces a hormone called adrenaline. This is the "fight" or "flight" response that is innate in animals and prepares them to either fight for their survival or run to save their lives. Adrenaline causes an increase in your breathing rate and also a rise in blood pressure and heart rate, which allows you to deal with dangerous/life-threatening situations in the short term. However, chronic exposure to this hormone, like that which results from the day-to-day stress of everyday life, can increase your risk for a heart attack.

Transcendental meditation has shown some promise in the prevention and treatment of coronary artery disease. It has been reported to decrease hypertension, atherosclerosis or cholesterol plaque buildup in vessels, and rates of smoking in patients with heart disease.

A recent study that was published in 2012 evaluated transcendental meditation in African Americans with heart disease. The study duration was five years. The study revealed that there was a 48% reduction in the rates of heart attack and stroke in those who practiced transcendental meditation on a regular basis when compared to their counterparts who attended a health education class during the same time period. Amazing results!

A statement from the American Heart Association suggests that transcendental meditation practice is the only meditation practice that has evidence for lowering blood pressure.

What is transcendental meditation?

Transcendental meditation usually involves the use of mantras to help move the mind from the physical day-to-day activities and helps settle the mind inwardly, into quieter levels of thought until you reach the most silent and peaceful level of your own consciousness. It is usually practiced twice a day for 15–20 minutes with your eyes closed. The use of mantras enables you to focus on the sound rather than the conceptual meaning, allowing the mind to transcend.

There are several different kinds of meditation techniques that are currently practiced. Examples of these include mindful meditation, which focuses on being in the present moment and being non-judgmental. Qigong meditation, a traditional Chinese form of meditation, that uses mantra and chanting and is a moving meditation technique which coordinates slow flowing movements of the body with deep rhythmic breathing into a calm meditative state of mind. It is a practice used to balance one's qi (chi) or what is called life balance. Lastly, devotional meditation, a form of Christian prayer, that is focused on making a connection to God.

Despite these different forms of meditation, transcendental meditation, again, is the only form of meditation that has been clinically shown to lower blood pressure.

Whereas transcendental meditation can be used as a way to lower stress levels and can reduce the risk for heart disease, you should bear in mind that it must be used as an adjunct or additional therapy and not as a replacement for lifestyle modification measures like healthy eating, exercising, quitting smoking, etc. For more on transcendental meditation, please visit their website at www.tm.org .

Medical management of hypertension:

When healthy lifestyle habits are not effective in reducing blood pressure, the next step is medication. To manage hypertension, one medication or a combination of different classes of medications can be tried until the correct dose and combination effective in lowering blood pressure with the fewest side effects is found. No two people are exactly alike in their response to medications, and no medication is completely without side effects, so there is usually an initial need for close follow-up until hypertension control is achieved. Hypertension medications work by reducing the amount of pressure on the arteries and the heart using different *mechanisms of action*. In the section below, I will simplify blood pressure medications into four broad categories based upon the medication's mechanism of action.

1. Medications that remove excess sodium and water from the body:

With less water or volume in the body, the amount of blood that has to be pumped by the heart is reduced. This change directly translates into reduced pressure in the blood vessels and therefore a reduced pressure that the heart has to pump against. These medications are usually referred to as "water pills" or diuretics. Examples include hydrochlorothiazide, furosemide, and spironolactone.

2. Medications that slow down the heart rate:

By slowing down the heart rate or by decreasing the number of times the heart beats each minute, the work load of the heart is reduced, which also decreases the blood pressure. Examples of these medications include beta-blockers like metoprolol and atenolol, and calcium channel blockers such as verapamil and diltiazem.

3. Medications that causes blood vessels to relax and dilate:

By relaxing and dilating the blood vessels or by preventing the vessels from tightening and constricting, blood can flow more easily and at a lower pressure. Medications that do this include the following:

a.) Angiotensin Converting Enzyme inhibitors (ACEI) like lisinopril and benazepril.
b.) Angiotensin II Receptor Blockers (ARB) like losartan and valsartan.
c.) Direct renin inhibitors like aliskiren.
d.) Vasodilators like hydralazine.

4. Medications that block hormones released under stress:

The hormones that are released when the body is under stress include epinephrine and norepinephrine. These hormones cause the heart rate to increase, resulting in narrowing of blood vessels. They also increase the force of contraction of the heart, leading to high blood pressure. Medications that block the effect of these stress hormones include the following:

a.) Alpha blockers like Cardura® (doxazosin mesylate).

b.) Alpha-beta blockers like carvedilol.

c.) Central acting agonists like clonidine.

Some may question why a person would take several medications which have side effects, just to prevent a disease that usually doesn't cause any symptoms. The answer is simple. Hypertension initially presents without symptoms, but if left untreated for prolonged periods of time, it can lead to serious, life-threatening complications (see fig. 10). All organs and systems in the body

Fig 10:

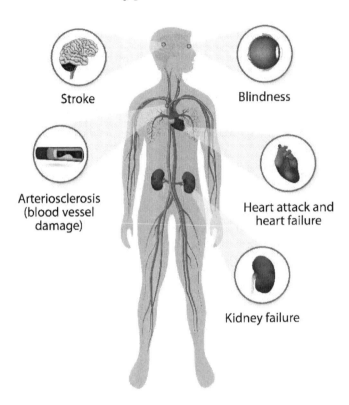

require a blood supply for oxygen and nutrients. This blood supply involves blood vessels that course throughout the entire body. As a result, hypertension can affect almost every organ system in the body, which can manifest clinically as a heart attack; a stroke; aneurysm formation, rupture and immediate death; blood clot formation; heart failure; kidney disease; loss of vision; trouble with memory or understanding; cardiac rhythm problems, like atrial fibrillation; loss of limbs; and the list goes on. Hypertension usually has no clinical signs in the beginning until some catastrophic event occurs like a stroke, which is usually irreversible. At this point, the only thing you can do is take medications to lower your blood pressure to prevent a second catastrophic incident from occurring. For this reason, hypertension is usually referred to as the "silent killer," and prompt diagnosis is vital to prevent these types of events.

Being diagnosed with hypertension may seem daunting at first, because so many facts are being thrown at you at once. Stop and take a deep breath. Remember that this is a chronic medical problem that will require LIFELONG changes to your everyday habits. You must take everything one step at a time and one day at a time. It is okay to ask lots of questions and make several follow-up appointments to see your provider until you have a clear understanding of what is happening and how to manage your condition. You should always share life-changing events in your life with your provider, such as a death in the family, divorce, job stress, etc., as these events may impact your health in a negative way and could make management of your blood pressure more difficult.

If you have done the absolute best you can to implement healthy lifestyle changes, but your blood pressure is still elevated, your provider may decide to begin medications to lower your blood pressure. It is always very important to take your medications as directed by your physician and be extremely honest about compliance with taking the medication.

Your provider will not be able to help you if he/she is unaware of whatever obstacles you face that act as barriers to you taking your medications as directed. It is also very important to have a blood pressure monitoring kit at home. At-home monitoring and regular follow-ups allow for early recognition of uncontrolled blood pressure, and can help with prompt management by your doctor. You and your doctor should develop a plan for at home monitoring in terms of the frequency, and what blood pressure recordings are considered emergent and would require that you either call the office or visit the emergency room or an urgent care center. It is important to realize that blood pressure fluctuates throughout the day, so you don't necessarily need to get "hung up" on one number. The goal is to have the majority of the recordings be within normal limits.

"Yesterday is not ours to recover, but tomorrow is ours to win or lose"

Lyndon B. Johnson

NOTES:

HIGH CHOLESTEROL

Grace is a 40-year-old female who is very health conscious. She exercises every day, doing at least one hour of aerobic activity, plus 30 minutes of strength training exercises. She has run several marathons and has competed in triathlons. She eats a heart healthy diet that has a high quantity of fruits and vegetables, whole grains, and is low in cholesterol and sodium. Grace has never smoked and does not drink any alcohol whatsoever. She denies having any chronic medical problems but does note a strong family history of heart attacks. Several of her family members have suffered from a heart attack at a young age, some in their mid-forties. Her adoption of a healthy lifestyle is a result of her strong family history of heart disease. She presents to her primary care physician for a routine follow up visit. After a thorough medical history, physical examination and laboratory testing, she is informed by her provider that she has high cholesterol. She is surprised by this diagnosis. After all, she leads a pretty healthy lifestyle.

She exercises rigorously, doesn't smoke or drink, and eats a very healthy diet, but her cholesterol is high. How can this be?

Cholesterol is a steroid alcohol (waxy fatlike substance) that is present naturally in all cells and body fluids. It is needed for the body to function normally. This substance is used by the body to produce different hormones like vitamin D. The body has two main sources of cholesterol. The first is from internal production by the liver. The second source of cholesterol is from ingestion. Eating foods high in cholesterol increases the total amount of cholesterol in the body. Cholesterol travels throughout the bloodstream in protein-covered particles called lipoproteins. Because cholesterol is an oily substance, it cannot travel efficiently in water (the bloodstream). The lipoprotein particle mixes better with the blood stream, allowing for transport. These protein particles contain cholesterol, triglycerides, and other components. Triglyceride is a fatty acid compound.

114

Cholesterol is carried in two kinds of particles in the blood: Low-density lipoproteins (LDL) and high-density lipoproteins (HDL). These different particles are named according to their ratio of fat-to-protein content, and therefore, their densities. For example, fat is less dense than protein, so a low-density lipoprotein (LDL) particle has a higher fat content than protein, while a high-density lipoprotein (HDL) particle has a higher protein content than fat. LDL is usually referred to as "bad" cholesterol. It transports cholesterol throughout the body. If your blood LDL levels are too high, the cholesterol contained within the particle is deposited in the walls of arteries, making them hard and stiff. Over time, as these cholesterol plaques build up in the artery walls, the artery narrows and eventually becomes completely occluded or blocked (see fig.11). This can lead to a heart attack, stroke, or other complications depending on the tissue that is supplied by the blocked artery.

HDL, on the other hand, contains more protein than cholesterol in its particle, and its job is to pick up the extra cholesterol in the arterial walls and take them back to the liver for breakdown and excretion. This is the reason that HDL is referred to as the "good" cholesterol. In addition to its role of cleaning up excess cholesterol, it also contains antioxidants that can be very beneficial to the blood vessels.

Fig. 11.

ARTERY DISEASE

ATHEROSCLEROSIS

BLOOD CLOT

STROKE   HEART ATTACK

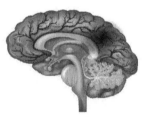 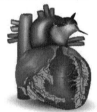

**BLOOD CLOT BLOCKS
BLOOD FLOW TO THE BRAIN**

**BLOOD CLOT BLOCKS
BLOOD FLOW TO THE HEART MUSCLE**

As mentioned earlier, the body makes all the cholesterol it needs, and it regulates the amount of cholesterol it produces based on the total amount of cholesterol in the body. The total amount of cholesterol in the body is determined by the amount ingested from food, plus the amount produced by the liver minus the amount excreted out of the body as waste products. If there is a high level of cholesterol in the blood, the body produces less cholesterol and excretes more, but if there is a low amount of cholesterol in the blood, the body makes more cholesterol and excretes less. This intricate mechanism used to balance out the total body cholesterol is an important concept to understand.

Patients like Beverly, who lead a very healthy lifestyle, including regular exercise, a lean diet, and no excess alcohol, CAN still have high blood levels of cholesterol. In Beverly's case, there could be a problem with one of the three mechanisms used to regulate total body cholesterol, or there may be an issue with some combination of all three mechanisms.

The most common abnormality is the overproduction of cholesterol by the liver, which is usually due to a genetic defect that is hereditary.

Nearly one in every two women in the US has high or borderline high cholesterol. The risk factors or causes of high cholesterol are the same factors that have been emphasized in other parts of the book, along with some factors that are unique to high cholesterol. These factors include the following:

- Cigarette smoking: Damages blood vessel walls, allowing for cholesterol deposition.
- Obesity: Predisposes patients to higher LDL levels.
- Poor diet: Diets high in saturated fats, trans-fats, and cholesterol.
- Large waist circumference: >35 inches in women.
- Physical inactivity: Increases LDL and lowers HDL.
- Diabetes: Damages blood vessel walls, allowing for cholesterol deposition.

- Heredity: Overproduction of LDL (bad) cholesterol.
- Alcohol: Excess alcohol ingestion leading to lower HDL levels.
- Gender and age: Premenopausal women usually have lower total cholesterol levels than postmenopausal women. As women age, their total cholesterol increases such that by age 50, women have higher total cholesterol levels than their male counterparts.

The American College of Cardiology guidelines recommend that your blood cholesterol profile be checked starting at age 20, and the check be repeated every 5 years. The blood test done to check your total body cholesterol requires that you fast, or not have anything to eat or drink, for 9-12 hours prior to having your blood drawn. We usually recommend that dinner should be your last meal, and then you should go to the laboratory first thing the next morning to get blood work done. This way, you are asleep for most of the fasting period, so you do not have to experience the discomfort of being hungry for a prolonged period of time.

Below is the list of cholesterol values.

Table 6

Desirable	Less than 200mg/dl
Borderline High	200-239mg/dl
High	240mg/dl and above

Table 7

LDL Cholesterol	
Optimal	Less than 100 mg/dl
Near/above optimal	100-129 mg/dl
Borderline high	130-159 mg/dl
High	160-189 mg/dl
Very high	190 mg/dl and over

If you have had a heart attack, stroke, diabetes or peripheral vascular disease, your LDL should be less than 70 mg/dl. Ask your doctor if you fall into this category.

Table 8

HDL Cholesterol	
High (optimal)	60 mg/dl
Low	Less than 40mg/dl

HDL of less than 50 mg/dl is considered low for women.

Table 9

Triglycerides	
Normal	Less than 150 mg/dl
Borderline high	150-199 mg/dl
High	200-499 mg/dl
Very high	500 mg/dl and above

Depending on risk factors, your doctor may recommend an optimal triglyceride level for you of less than 100 mg/dl.

High cholesterol, like hypertension, has no symptoms, but if it goes untreated, it can put you at high risk for a cardiovascular event. For example, if cholesterol builds up in the walls of the blood vessels, it causes the blood vessel to narrow to the point where you either get minimal or no blood flow to the organ and tissue supplied by the vessel. If this is one of the blood vessels of the heart, this narrowing can manifest clinically as chest pains and pressure, or what is called "angina." If it occurs in the blood vessels of the leg, it can cause pain with activity that is relieved with rest called "claudication."

Cholesterol plaques in the vessel can be very unstable and prone to rupture, even when the plaque is not causing any significant occlusion to the vessel, and therefore no limitation to blood flow and no symptoms. With this hemodynamically   insignificant occlusion, patients have no symptoms and are unaware of the high risk for rupture. When it does rupture, the body's clotting system is activated, resulting in rapid clot formation and complete occlusion of the blood vessel or artery, causing an acute heart attack. This clot can break off and travel to another set of blood vessels such as those in the brain, causing a stroke. This blockage can happen anywhere in the body, and can involve any organ system in the body. This all means that you do not need to have the arteries of your heart 70% occluded or greater to cause a heart attack, minimal and clinically insignificant blood vessel narrowing of about 30% can cause an acute heart attack if the cholesterol plaques in the blood vessel walls are unstable. Cholesterol plaques that can rupture are referred to as vulnerable cholesterol plaques. Vulnerable plaques are at least as important for causing a heart attack as coronary arteries with narrowing greater than or equal to 70%. Vulnerable plaques and plaque rupture are one of the reasons why a person can have no warning signs before sustaining a massive heart attack. If you have blockages in the blood vessels of your heart that are greater than or equal to 70%, you will often have clinical signs of chest discomfort, which worsens with activity and improves with rest. This can serve as a clue that there is a problem with your heart, and it will cause you to seek medical care sooner. A vulnerable plaque, on the other hand, gives no clinical signs prior to acutely rupturing and causing a significant event. These abnormal arteries are not usually picked up by the conventional stress test, so even with a negative stress test, you are not at zero risk of having a cardiovascular event.

How do we prevent cholesterol plaque rupture and an acute heart attack, especially for minimally occluded vessels? By lowering total body cholesterol.

First-line treatment for high cholesterol involves lifestyle modifications that include diets low in saturated fats and cholesterol. The TLC diet, mentioned in the section on diet, has been shown to decrease LDL cholesterol and increase HDL cholesterol. Other lifestyle changes include exercise, weight loss, smoking cessation, moderate alcohol intake, and controlling other cardiac risk factors like hypertension and diabetes. If your cholesterol levels continue to be elevated despite these modifications, then your provider may recommend starting medication.

There are several medications on the market today for lowering LDL cholesterol. The most popular and effective of these medications are called statins. Some examples of statin medications include atorvastatin, simvastatin, rosuvastatin, and pravastatin. Statins work by decreasing the body's production of LDL, and increasing the liver's ability to remove it from the blood. Statins have been shown to lower LDL cholesterol by 20-60%. They also decrease triglycerides and increase HDL. These types of drugs usually take effect in 6-8 weeks. While on statin therapy, your liver function should be monitored with some regularity. Alcohol consumption should be avoided, because the liver is involved in metabolizing these medications.

It is known that the beneficial effects of statins in preventing cardiovascular events go beyond preventing plaque buildup in blood vessels. Statins have other beneficial effects that are unrelated to their mechanism of action. These effects are called "pleiotropic effects," which means they produce more than one effect and can include benefits like anti-inflammatory properties, antioxidant properties, and increased nitric oxide availability, which allow the blood vessels to relax and dilate. These and other effects contribute to the influence of statins in enabling a normal and healthy functioning heart.

Most people tolerate statins quite well. A rare side effect that needs to be monitored while taking statin medications daily is muscle breakdown. This can be a very severe side effect. Muscle breakdown (statin myopathy) usually manifests as muscle pain and in severe cases can cause or present with dark-colored urine. This tea-colored urine results from the breakdown products from damaged muscle cells that are released into the bloodstream. If these symptoms develop, you should notify your health care provider immediately and proceed to the emergency room. When taking statins, you should also be careful about eating foods like grapefruit, as they increase the potency of statins and therefore raise the risk of side effects.

Ezetimibe is another class of cholesterol-lowering drugs that prevent the body from absorbing cholesterol from food. This medication lowers LDL and may lower triglycerides and raise HDL. It is still unclear from studies whether this drug decreases the risk of heart attacks and strokes.

Bile acid sequestrants are another class of cholesterol lowering drugs that work by binding bile acids in the intestine and preventing them from being reabsorbed. Bile acids are steroid acids made in the liver using cholesterol. These bile acids travel to the intestine, where they aid in the absorption of dietary fats. When bile acids are bound in the intestine and removed from the body, the total amount of cholesterol in the body is lowered, because bile acids are made from cholesterol. The body has to maintain a certain level of bile acids in order to enable digestion. When the bile acids are not reabsorbed and the amount in the blood decreases, the liver must produce more bile acids to maintain a certain amount in the body. The liver then uses the cholesterol in the body to make bile acids.

Bile acid sequestrants medications bind bile acids in the intestine and cause them to be removed as waste, and not reabsorbed back into the blood stream. This lowers the total amount of bile acids in the body and the liver has to make more to maintain normal body levels of bile acids. As a result, cholesterol is diverted for the production of bile acids, which lowers total body cholesterol. This class of medications can also produce the side effects of stomach upset, nausea, bloating, and cramping. Examples of this class of drugs include cholestyramine, colestipole, and colesevelam. These medications can lower mild to moderately elevated LDL. Because these drugs only cause a modest decrease in LDL cholesterol, they are not typically the first-line agents used in treating high cholesterol.

Fibrates are another class of cholesterol-lowering medications used to lower triglycerides and raise HDL, but they have little to no effect on LDL. Examples of these drugs include gemfibrozil and fenofibrate. Like statins, these medications can also cause muscle breakdown (myopathy).

Nicotinic acids or niacin is usually added as a second drug in patients whose cholesterol panel is still not optimal despite being on the maximum tolerable dose of a statin. Its major side effects include flushing, which can be overcome by taking an aspirin 30 minutes prior to taking niacin.

Other nutritional supplements that have beneficial effects on lowering cholesterol include omega-3-fatty acids, garlic, and soy protein.

Once you are on cholesterol-lowering medications, your target goal for LDL depends on your risk factors for developing heart disease. The heart disease risk is determined based on your Framingham risk score, which is a calculation used to determine your 10-year risk for coronary heart disease. You should talk to your doctor about the Framingham score and goal LDL numbers for you. Once your LDL goal is reached, you will remain on the medication combination and dose that got you to your goal LDL and will probably stay on the medications and dose indefinitely. You will also be required to have blood testing one to two times a year to monitor your liver function while on these medications.

"You can't cross the sea merely by standing and staring at the water."

Rabindranath Tagore

NOTES:

DIABETES MELLITUS

Heather is a 55-year-old female who was recently diagnosed with type 2 diabetes mellitus. She has begun to monitor blood sugars at home. Her blood sugars have been relatively well controlled on the two medications that her primary care provider prescribed for her. She has taken her medications religiously every day. Heather has a strong family history of diabetes and heart disease. She reports a hand full of relatives who have passed away in their mid to late fifties from complications of diabetes as well as heart disease. This information is very disturbing to her, and she would like to know what her risk for having a heart attack is, given her current medical illness and strong family history of heart disease.

As of 2014, there are an estimated 387 million people with diabetes worldwide. Type 2 diabetes accounts for about 90% of all diabetes cases. From 2012-2014, diabetes was responsible for an estimated 1.5-4.9 million deaths each year. The number of people with diabetes is expected to increase to 592 billion by 2035.

Heart disease along with concomitant or associated diabetes mellitus is more serious in women than in men. When evaluating gender differences regarding long-term outcomes in patients who have diabetes mellitus and have suffered a heart attack, a few observations can be made. Women with diabetes mellitus generally have a lower survival rate after suffering a cardiovascular event than their male counterparts with similar medical conditions. Women also end up with a poorer quality of life than males who have similar medical illnesses. Diabetes doubles a person's risk of death. The rate of death from diabetes in women between the ages of 25 and 44 years is more than three times the rate of death in women without diabetes.

Diabetes mellitus is a lifelong disease state that is characterized by high blood sugar (also known as glucose) levels. Glucose is an important source of energy for tissues and organs in the body; and for large and vital organs like the brain, it is the main source of energy. The body has two major sources of glucose. The first source is from internal production by the liver and the second is from the food we ingest. There is a small organ in the body that lies right below the stomach called the pancreas, which produces a hormone called insulin. Insulin is very important because it allows organs and tissues to extract glucose from the blood and use it for energy. Without insulin, tissues are unable to obtain and utilize glucose, and the glucose remains in the bloodstream, producing high levels of blood sugar. Over time, high blood glucose can cause damage to all the organs and systems in the body. More specifically, it affects the heart, kidney, nervous system, and the eyes, resulting in heart attacks, kidney failure, strokes, nerve damage, and blindness.

There are three main types of diabetes: type 1 diabetes, type 2 diabetes, and gestational diabetes. There is also another category of diabetes called Mature Onset Diabetes of the Young (MODY), that accounts for less than 5% of all individuals diagnosed with diabetes. This category of diabetes will not be covered in this book.

Type 1 diabetes is usually referred to as insulin-dependent diabetes. It usually occurs in childhood and was once called juvenile onset diabetes. This type of diabetes arises when the pancreas either produces very little or no insulin. For an unknown reason, the body's immune system attacks and destroys the pancreas, resulting in little to no production of insulin. As a result, treatment of this type of diabetes always involves insulin injections, as these patients make minimal to no insulin. Type 1 diabetes accounts for only 5-10% of all diabetes and may have some hereditary predilection or predisposition.

Type 2 diabetes is the most common form of diabetes. It used to be referred to as adult onset diabetes, but with the rapid rise in obesity, especially in teenagers, type 2 diabetes is now also seen in young people.

Type 2 diabetes is characterized both by the pancreas' underproduction of insulin and by the body's resistance to the insulin already produced by the pancreas. With this disease, tissues and organs in the body require more insulin than normal to extract glucose from the blood because they do not respond to normal levels of insulin. In the early stages of the disease process, treatment of type 2 diabetes involves the use of medications that either increase the tissue and organ sensitivity to insulin so that less insulin is required by the body, or decrease the liver's glucose production, lowering the overall blood glucose levels. Lifestyle habits and genetics have a bigger effect on type 2 diabetes, and obesity is a major risk factor for the development of type 2 diabetes. People who are genetically predisposed to having the disease may not manifest diabetes until they become obese, at which time the diabetes becomes evident. Along with obesity, a lack of exercise and a poor diet also contribute to the clinical manifestation of type 2 diabetes.

Gestational diabetes is usually diagnosed in the middle of or late in pregnancy in women who do not have a history of diabetes. Its incidence, according to the National Institute of Health, is 2-10% of all pregnancies, and it often resolves once the pregnancy ends. Approximately 5-10% of women with gestational diabetes go on to develop diabetes in the future. Most often, these patients end up with type 2 diabetes many years after giving birth. Gestational diabetes is very similar to type 2 diabetes in that it develops when the organs and tissues of the body are resistant to insulin. As a result, gestational diabetes patients require higher levels of insulin for the organs and tissues to adequately extract glucose from the blood, just like in type 2 diabetic patients.

The risk factors for developing gestational diabetes are also similar to type 2 diabetes, and they include: obesity prior to pregnancy, having a diagnosis of pre-diabetes prior to pregnancy, a family history of diabetes, giving birth to a child who weighs more than nine pounds or giving birth to a stillborn, and lastly, being from a high risk ethnic group like African Americans, Hispanics, Asians, or Native Americans. Gestational diabetes is unique in that not only does high blood glucose affect the mother, the glucose also crosses the placenta and affects the fetus. The high levels of glucose that the fetus is exposed to cause an increase in insulin production. Insulin stimulates growth, causing the fetus's body to grow larger than normal. Exposure to excessive amounts of blood sugar will increases the risk of fetal distress, abnormal development of the fetal organs, and sometimes death. Gestational diabetes often leads to early labor induction and a higher chance of a caesarean delivery.

Symptoms of diabetes mellitus:

The symptoms of type 2 diabetes usually take some time to manifest, so you can have the disease for many years before you start to show symptoms. Type 1 diabetes usually produces symptoms a lot sooner. The classic symptoms of diabetes include increased thirst (polydipsia), frequent urination (polyuria), and increased hunger (polyphagia). With high concentrations of glucose in the blood, fluid is pulled out of the cells and into the blood vessels. This movement of fluid out of the cells causes the cells to become dehydrated, which manifests clinically as increased thirst and urination. Tissues and organs are unable to extract glucose from the blood for energy, which triggers an intense hunger. The patient eats more, but this turns out to be futile, because the tissues and organs are not able to extract the glucose. The body resorts to using alternative fuel sources for energy, such as muscles and stored fat. The breakdown of these alternative fuel sources causes weight loss. However, this is not a good way to lose weight because you are losing protein and muscle mass. The weight loss is also accompanied by other symptoms, like chronic fatigue, lightheadedness, nausea, vomiting, and feeling hot and cold at inappropriate times.

Most of the symptoms associated with diabetes mellitus are non-life threatening, except in two instances. The first serious complication of diabetes mellitus occurs when the blood sugar gets too high, as in the cases of diabetic ketoacidosis (seen mostly in type 1 diabetes) and hyperosmolar coma (seen mostly in type 2 diabetes). The second serious complication of diabetes happens when blood sugar levels fall too low, which is called hypoglycemia. These two life threatening complications usually require treatment in the intensive care unit.

Complications of diabetes mellitus:

Diabetes mellitus can lead to many complications if it is not treated. The long-term complications of diabetes are listed below:

- **Heart disease**: Diabetes destroys the blood vessels of the heart, leading to heart attacks. Death rates from heart disease are higher in adults with diabetes than in those without. Studies show mortality rates as high as 1.7 times in diabetics when compared to non-diabetics. Diabetes also increases the risk of developing hypertension, which can complicate heart disease.

- **Kidney failure**: Diabetes can destroy the blood vessels in the kidney, leading to the need for dialysis or even a kidney transplant. Diabetes is the most common cause of kidney failure in the US. It is reported that 44% of new cases of kidney failure are in diabetics.

- **Blindness:** Diabetes can lead to many eye problems, including glaucoma, cataracts, and even blindness. It remains the number one cause of blindness in the US in people 20-74 years old.

- **Nerve damage:** Also called neuropathy, nerve damage manifests as numbness and tingling in the tips of the hands and feet that then spreads upwards. Neuropathy can include a burning and painful sensation in the hands and feet. Over time, diabetic neuropathy can lead to the loss of all sense of feeling in the hands and feet. Losing all feeling in the legs can lead to complications like non-healing ulcers, foot fractures, and serious infections that can eventually require amputation. 60-70% of diabetics have some form of nerve damage or neuropathy. Diabetes can affect any and all nerves in the body, leading to problems that are specific to the affected organs. For example, damage to nerves in the gastrointestinal tract can lead to digestion problems like nausea, vomiting, and slow transit time of food in the GI tract. Nerve damage to sexual organs can contribute to erectile dysfunction in men.

- **Cognitive deficits:** Studies have shown some linkage between diabetes and a decline in brain function, like in Alzheimer's disease. More extensive studies still need to be done to prove a linkage between these two illnesses.

- **Skin complications:** Diabetics are prone to skin infections and other diabetic related skin disorders that cause skin discolorations, rashes, and blisters.

Making the diagnosis of diabetes:

The diagnosis of diabetes is usually made with blood testing since most patients are asymptomatic in the early stages of the disease. These blood tests include the hemoglobin A1c (HbA1c), fasting plasma glucose test (FPG), and oral glucose tolerance test (OGTT).

HbA1c is used for the diagnosis of type 2 diabetes. The HbA1c value is a reflection of a person's average blood sugar levels over a three-month period. This test does not usually require the patient to fast to be accurate. The value is usually obtained as a percentage, and a diagnosis of diabetes requires that the percentage be greater than or equal to 6.5% (see table 10). A fasting plasma glucose test (FPG) requires several hours of fasting and is most accurate when performed in the morning. An FPG of 126 mg/dl is the definition of diabetes (see table 10). An oral glucose tolerance test (OGTT) is a somewhat more intensive test than the FPG. It requires an eight-hour fast prior to testing. You will be asked to drink a sugar water drink containing 75 grams of glucose. Blood is drawn before ingestion of the sugar water drink and then 1 hour, 2 hours, and 3 hours after you consume the sugar drink. A glucose level of 200 mg/dl two hours after ingestion of the sugar water is diagnostic of diabetes (see table 11). The OGTT is used to screen for gestational diabetes. Keep in mind that all these tests have to be repeated at least twice on different days before a definitive diagnosis of diabetes can be made.

Sometimes a random glucose level can be drawn at the doctor's office to make the diagnosis. A random glucose level over 200 mg/dl along with symptoms of diabetes (frequent urination, thirst, and weight loss without another explanation) confirms a diagnosis of diabetes.

Table 10:

Diagnosis	HbA1c (%)	FPGT (mg/dl)	OGTT (2hr post mg/dl)
Normal	≤ 5.6	≤ 99	≤ 139
Prediabetes	5.7 – 6.4	100-125	140 - 199
Diabetes	≥ 6.5	≥ 126	≥ 200

Table 11:

OGTT for diagnosis of gestational diabetes

Time after sugar water ingestion	OGTT (mg/dl)
Before	≥ 99
1-hour after	≥ 180
2 hours' after	≥ 155
3 hours' after	≥ 140

Treatment:

The goals of diabetes treatment are to avoid the long-term, chronic complications of diabetes as well as to prevent the day-to-day struggles with too high a blood sugar level (hyperglycemia), and too low a blood sugar level (hypoglycemia). The initial treatment for type 2 and gestational diabetes includes changes in lifestyle habits, as we have discussed throughout this book, including weight loss, increased physical activity, a healthy diet, and smoking cessation. Weight loss and exercise increase the tissues' and organs' sensitivity to insulin.

Despite these changes in lifestyle, you may still have high blood sugar levels and require medications to lower your blood sugar. If oral medications in combination are not adequately maintaining blood sugar levels, then insulin injections can be added for better blood sugar control.

Type 1 diabetic patients require insulin injections as the initial treatment because the pancreas, the organ responsible for producing the insulin that the body needs, has failed and therefore produces little to no insulin. Insulin, is therefore the first line therapy for these patients. Lifestyle changes should also be implemented.

There are several classes of diabetes medications, which are categorized based on their mechanism of action. These include:

- Sulfonylureas (glyburide, glimepiride, glipizide): This class functions by stimulating the pancreas to release insulin. Side effects include weight gain, and hypoglycemia.
- Biguanides (metformin): This medication improves the insulin sensitivity of tissues and organs, as well as inhibiting the release of glucose from the liver. Biguanides can also decrease levels of LDL (or bad cholesterol) and cause some weight loss.
- Thiazolidinediones (rosiglitazone, pioglitazone): These work by preventing the liver from releasing glucose, and also

by improving the insulin sensitivity of tissues and organs. However, these medications can cause a heart attack or heart failure and therefore should not be used in adults with heart or kidney problems.

- Meglitinides (repaglinide, nateglinide): These drugs work by stimulating the pancreas to release insulin.

- Dipeptidyl-peptidase 4 (DPP-4) inhibitors (sitagliptin, linagliptin, saxagliptin): These medications prevent the liver from releasing glucose and stimulate insulin release from the pancreas. They do not cause weight gain.

- Alpha-glucosidase inhibitors (acarbose, miglitol): slow down the breakdown of starches. The side effects include abdominal gas and stomach pain, but they do not cause weight gain.

- Bile acid sequestrants (colesevelam): This class of drugs was mentioned previously in the cholesterol section. They not only lower cholesterol, but can also lower blood sugar when used with other diabetic medications. The side effects of these medications include abdominal gas and constipation.

• Sodium-glucose transporter 2 (SGLT2) inhibitors (canagliflozin, dapagliflozin, empagliflozin): This class of medications works by preventing the kidneys from reabsorbing glucose, so glucose is eliminated in the urine. This class can potentially cause vaginal yeast infections.

• Amylin mimetics (pramlintide): These medications are administered via injection and are used along with insulin. They also stimulate the release of insulin. These medications can cause some weight loss, and side effects include stomach upset.

• Incretin mimetics (exenatide, liraglutide): These are also administered via injection and are used with sulfonylureas. They work by stimulating insulin release and can cause some weight loss.

- Insulin: This is, of course, given as an injection. There are many short-acting and long-acting forms. Your physician will recommend which one is best for you.

Please consult the package inserts of each medication for more extensive details about these drugs.

Who should be screened for diabetes?

Type 1 diabetes patients generally present with overt symptoms of diabetes at a young age, so screening is usually not necessary for this group. Type 2 diabetes presents more gradually over a period of several years and therefore can be detected and treated early in the course of the disease process before definite symptoms occur. The general recommendation is that screening should be done in anyone above 45 years of age, using any of the tests mentioned above. If the screening is negative, then screening every three years is recommended. If the test diagnoses a person as pre-diabetic, then the test should be repeated in a year along with implementation of lifestyle changes. If the patient is younger than 45 years of age, screening is recommended in those whose BMI is higher than 25 as well as those with additional risk factors, like high cholesterol, high blood pressure, no physical activity, and/or giving birth to a baby 9 pounds and over.

Once you have been given a diagnosis of diabetes, it is important to monitor your blood sugar at home to see how well it is being controlled. Glucose meters for home monitoring can be purchased. You will be given instructions on when to check your blood sugar, but it is generally checked both before and after meals and before bedtime. All results should be recorded and reviewed with the health care provider. These numbers will dictate how food, medication, stress, and activity affect your blood sugar. Talk with your doctor about what your goals should be, but in general, blood glucose should be between 70 and 130 mg/dl before a meal and less than 180 mg/dl one to two hours after eating.

Managing diabetes may seem very frustrating and overwhelming, but if taken one day at a time along with a management plan, a relatively normal lifestyle can be enjoyed. Taking all your medications, filling your prescriptions on time to avoid missing doses, and monitoring your blood sugars, will result in a rewarding improvement in blood glucose and HbA1c numbers.

"The time is always right to do what is right"

Martin Luther King, Jr

NOTES:

METABOLIC SYNDROME

Metabolic syndrome is a syndrome defined by having any three of these five conditions:

- High blood pressure
- High blood glucose
- Abdominal obesity (waist circumference >35 inches)
- High triglyceride
- Low HDL (good cholesterol)

Metabolic syndrome increases your risk of developing cardiovascular disease. Having any one of these conditions individually, increases your risk of having a cardiovascular event. Having three or more concurrently, increases your risk even further. Among patients with a diagnosis of heart disease, approximately 50% have metabolic syndrome. Among patients with premature heart disease, approximately 37% will be diagnosed with metabolic syndrome. The good news is that heart disease can be prevented, or its progression can be slowed by the same measures that have been described throughout this book, including aggressive lifestyle changes. The prevalence of metabolic syndrome is growing because of the rise in obesity in recent years, and it will soon surpass smoking as the leading risk factor for heart disease.

"What you do today can improve all your tomorrows".

Ralph Marston

NOTES:

Hormone replacement therapy and risk for cardiovascular events.

Hormone replacement therapy (HRT) is a treatment given to postmenopausal women and includes either estrogen alone, or estrogen with progesterone. Progesterone is usually prescribed to women who still have their uterus. This is to prevent an increased risk of endometrial cancer associated with giving estrogen alone. HRT helps with the short-term side effects of menopause like hot flashes, vaginal dryness, dry skin, sleeplessness, and bladder irritation. It also has other long-term beneficial effects, like decreasing the risk of osteoporosis in a population in which the risk of osteoporosis is high. HRT also reduces the risk of colon cancer and possibly decreases the incidence of Alzheimer's disease. HRT makes blood vessels less stiff and more pliable, allowing the blood to flow through them freely.

At the same time, HRT is not without its share of risk. It is associated with an increased incidence of endometrial cancer in women with their uterus still intact, who receive estrogen without progesterone. HRT is also associated with an increased risk of breast cancer, blood clots, strokes, and cardiovascular disease, including heart attacks. We know that women's risk for heart disease is usually lower than that for men in a similar age group before menopause. But as women age and their estrogen levels decrease, their risk for heart disease increases.

Because of this association of decreased estrogen levels and an increased risk for heart disease, expert panels recommended HRT therapy for *all* menopausal women in the late 1980s and early 1990s! Recent studies like the Women's Health Initiative (WHI) and the Heart and Estrogen/Progesterone Replacement Study (HERS) have not necessarily corroborated this hypothesis. Instead, the WHI study showed that women who began HRT many years after menopause had an increased risk of developing a cardiovascular event, and breast cancer. Follow up studies, however, have suggested that this increased risk of cardiovascular events might be related to age and the cardiovascular risk assessment of the patient at the start of the HRT. In other words, patients with risk factors for heart disease are at higher risk for a cardiovascular event if they decide to take HRT. Whereas, younger patients who have minimal to no risk factors for cardiovascular events may not have an increased risk of heart disease with HRT.

A guideline committee has attempted to summarize these study findings that sometimes seem to contradict one other. The recommendations from this committee are as follows: If you have a history of a heart attack, stroke, and blood clots, you should not take HRT, as your risk for a cardiovascular event is high. If a woman is already on HRT, the decision to continue or discontinue the medication should be discussed at length with her doctor and should be left at her and her doctor's discretion. However, if a woman develops a cardiovascular event *while* on HRT, then the medication needs to be stopped immediately!

If you absolutely must take some form of hormone replacement due to intolerable side effects of menopause, you should take the lowest effective dose possible for the shortest amount of time needed for treatment. Alternatively, you can take other forms of estrogen that have a restricted amount of systemic or whole body absorption, such as a vaginal estrogen preparation either in a cream, tablet, or ring form.

There is some evidence that younger women with minimal to no cardiovascular risk factors may not be at increased risk of a cardiovascular event with HRT, and there might even be some cardiovascular benefit if HRT is started close to the beginning of menopause. More studies are still needed to further corroborate this.

Overall, lifestyle changes like exercise, a healthy diet, quitting smoking, and controlling blood pressure, cholesterol, and blood glucose are recommended to reduce the risk of cardiovascular disease in menopausal women.

"A desire to be in charge of our own lives, a need for control, is born in each of us. It is essential to our mental health, and our success, that we take control"

Robert Foster Bennett

NOTES:

Aspirin for the prevention of heart attack in women

Aspirin has been shown to have many beneficial effects in men with heart disease. It decreases the inflammatory process associated with heart attack and inhibits blood clot formation. A heart attack happens when unstable cholesterol plaques in the arteries of the heart rupture and a blood clot forms that completely obstructs the artery and prevents blood from delivering oxygen and nutrients to the heart. Aspirin can block this process and reduce the risk of heart attack, stroke, and death. Aspirin also has some side effects that can be detrimental. It can cause stomach ulcers, intestinal bleeding, and bleeding elsewhere, such as in the brain.

The landmark trials that have examined aspirin and its role in the prevention of heart attack mainly included male participants. Many have wondered if aspirin has the same effect in female patients. A trial called the *Women's Health Study* sought to answer this question. It enrolled 40,000 women in the study. Overall, the study showed that aspirin prevented heart attacks and strokes in women over the age of 65 years to the same degree that it did in men. The recommended dose of aspirin is 81 mg daily, or 100 mg every other day. In women younger than 65 years of age, there was a small benefit to taking aspirin, but there was a higher risk of bleeding complications in this age group of women that far outweighed the benefit of aspirin.

What we do know for sure is that if a woman is having a heart attack, taking an aspirin (81 - 162 mg chewable aspirin) decreases her chance of dying from that heart attack. Also, if you have had a heart attack or stroke in the past, taking a baby aspirin does decrease your chances of dying from another cardiovascular event. It is well known that your risk for having a second heart attack increases after your first one.

Also, if you do have evidence of partial artery blockage in your heart that manifests as chest pains or angina, then a baby aspirin can prevent you from having a heart attack.

However, if you are a relatively healthy woman who is younger than 65 years of age with no heart disease, the bleeding risk from taking a baby aspirin far outweighs the benefit of preventing a heart attack, and the guidelines do not generally recommend routine usage of aspirin in this group. If you are under 65 years of age and are unsure of your risk and whether or not you would benefit from daily baby aspirin use, you should have a discussion with your primary care physician to weigh the risks and benefits of chronic aspirin use as it pertains to your risk for a cardiovascular event.

"I believe that the greatest gift you can give your family and the world is a healthy you".

Joyce Meyer

NOTES:

ANTIOXIDANTS

What are antioxidants? Antioxidants are vitamins and minerals like vitamin E, vitamin C, and beta-carotene that are found in food sources. Antioxidants are beneficial to human health because they can prevent disease. The many cells in the human body require energy to function normally. This energy is derived from food sources. The byproduct left over after the conversion of food to energy is a substance called oxygen free radicals. Oxygen free radicals cause damage to all cells in the body. In terms of heart disease, oxygen free radicals make LDL cholesterol more likely to build up as plaques on the walls of arteries. Antioxidants prevent these free radicals from causing destruction to cells. Because of the beneficial effects of antioxidants, antioxidant supplements were studied to determine whether there were any cardiovascular benefits from taking them. The conclusion of these studies that examined the effect of antioxidants like beta-carotene, vitamin E, and vitamin C on women was that they are ineffective in reducing heart attacks, strokes, or death from any cardiovascular cause. These studies have led to the general recommendation that antioxidant supplements not be used for primary or secondary prevention of a cardiovascular event.

Although antioxidant supplements showed no benefit, foods rich in antioxidants, like dark green, red, and orange vegetables and fruits, along with whole grains have been shown to reduce the risk of cardiovascular events. It is not entirely clear why the supplements showed no cardiovascular benefit, yet some cardiovascular benefit was seen when the antioxidants were obtained from a food source. One proposed theory is that the cardiovascular benefits seen in antioxidants obtained from a food source may have to do with other nutrients like lycopenes and flavonoids that are also contained in these foods in their natural state which are not present in the supplement form. These nutrients may work alongside the antioxidants and are most likely the source of any cardiovascular benefit.

"It is health that is real wealth and not pieces of gold and silver".

Mahatma Gandhi

NOTES:

HEART ATTACK

Irene is a 45-year-old female who has had diabetes and hypertension for about five years. Her blood pressure has been well controlled, but her blood sugars have been a bit more of a challenge. She has been having some chest discomfort, which she described as a burning sensation in the middle of her chest which radiates down to her stomach. She thought her symptoms were from indigestion or heartburn, as she's had similar symptoms in the past. Irene has taken antacids for her heartburn in the past and felt that it relieved her symptoms. She decided to take antacids for her current symptoms.

Initially, there was some improvement, but over several days, her symptoms intensified. She found herself taking whole bottles of antacids with only minimal improvement in the discomfort. One night, her symptoms became so severe that she decided to drive to the emergency room. She was initially treated for gastroesophageal reflux disease (GERD) with a gastrointestinal (GI) cocktail because she insisted to the physicians in the ER that her symptoms were identical to heartburn episodes in the past, only more intense. Since she experienced minimal relief with the GI cocktail, an electrocardiogram and lab work were ordered. The electrocardiogram showed that Irene was having a heart attack. She was rushed to the catheterization laboratory, where she underwent an angiogram. A cardiac angiogram is when contrast dye visible to x-ray is injected into the arteries of the heart. The x-ray images show the dye as it flows into the vessels and identifies blockages in the major arteries that supply the heart.

Irene's angiogram revealed that one of her major arteries that supplies blood to the largest proportion of the heart was almost completely blocked. This artery, when completely blocked acutely, is often referred to as the "widow maker", as patients rarely survive a sudden occlusion of this vessel. She then immediately underwent cardiac bypass surgery. Because Irene had waited several days before seeking medical attention, her outcome was poor. Irene had sustained a lot of tissue damage to her heart that was irreversible because of the length of time that passed before seeking help. She survived that hospital stay but sustained disabilities that affect her quality of life.

<u>Heart attack symptoms</u>

When people think about the symptoms of a heart attack, the image that comes to mind is that of a man with a look of agony on his face, and his left hand clutching his chest. While this is considered the classic presentation of a heart attack, it is usually not the case for women. You remember our story of Angie, the hard working single Mom in the first section of this book.

Because their symptoms are not classic, women often fail to recognize that they are having a cardiac event. When women do eventually present to the emergency room late in the disease process, the diagnosis is often either delayed or missed entirely, leading to higher morbidity and mortality levels in women compared to men with similar clinical characteristics who present with the classic signs of a heart attack. The symptoms of a heart attack include the following:

- Chest discomfort, which is usually described as a squeezing, pressure-like pain in the center of the chest. The pressure has been described as "an elephant sitting on my chest." The pressure lasts for more than a few minutes, and it can be intermittent.
- The chest pain or discomfort can radiate to the arms (usually the left arm, but it can radiate to both) or to the back, neck, and stomach. Stomach discomfort usually is mistaken for heartburn or acid reflux.
- There is usually difficulty catching one's breath or shortness of breath associated with the chest discomfort.
- Other symptoms include breaking out in a cold sweat, feeling anxious, and

having a sense of doom,
lightheadedness, nausea, and vomiting.

Although chest discomfort is the most common symptom of a heart attack in men, fewer than 30% of women report that they experienced chest pain with their heart attack. Forty-three percent of women did not have any chest discomfort at any time during their event. Women's symptoms tend to be subtle, and they generally experience these symptoms up to a month prior to having a heart attack. In a study performed by the National Institutes of Health (NIH) that examined women's symptoms prior to a heart attack, it was found that 70% of women complained of unusual fatigue, 48% had sleep disturbances, 42% reported shortness of breath, 39% complained of indigestion, and 35% experienced anxiety. During their heart attack, 58% of women had shortness of breath, 55% complained of weakness, 43% felt unusual fatigue, 39% reported a cold sweat, and 39% experienced dizziness.

Again, the symptoms of a heart attack can be quite subtle for women. It may begin with nonspecific symptoms that occur up to a month in advance, but a heart attack can also be abrupt and simply produce the most excruciating chest pains/pressure that a person has ever experienced. Symptom presentation varies from woman to woman. It is important to know the signs and symptoms of a heart attack so that you can seek medical attention promptly if you experience any of the signs. When several of these symptoms are present at the same time, the chance that you are having a heart attack increases. You should *not* downplay the symptoms, and you should *not* wait for more than five minutes before calling 911 or another emergency medical service for help. The same applies when you suspect someone else may be having a heart attack. Do not wait more than five minutes before calling 911. If your area does not provide emergency medical services, get someone to drive you to the emergency room. Avoid driving yourself to the emergency room unless, you have no other choice.

"He who has health, has hope; and he who has hope has everything".

Thomas Carlyl

NOTES:

CONCLUSION

I hope this book has been very helpful in educating you on heart disease, the risk factors associated with heart disease, and how you can prevent a heart attack. I also hope that you are now familiar with the signs and symptoms of a heart attack so that you can recognize the symptoms earlier and seek medical attention IMMEDIATELY.

Remember: **Time is tissue**! The quicker you recognize your symptoms, the sooner you'll seek medical attention. Ultimately, the faster you receive medical intervention, the more of your precious heart tissue you will save. Timely treatment goes a long way in reducing the high percentage of morbidity and mortality caused by heart disease that is seen in women.

Take care of yourself. You cannot be an effective caretaker of others if you are not healthy yourself.

The take-home points about this book are summarized below:

Heart disease is preventable using the following measures:

- Quit smoking.
- Eat a healthy diet.
- Consume alcohol in moderation or none at all.
- Exercise regularly.
- Maintain a healthy weight.
- Maintain optimal blood pressure, blood sugar, and cholesterol levels.
- Schedule regular appointments with your provider.
- Know the warning signs of a heart attack, and call 911 no later than five minutes after you suspect you are having a heart attack.

I would like to thank you for your interest in this book. I wish you all the best. Here is to your good health and a long and happy life!

"It's in the reach of my arms

The span of my hips,

The stride of my step,

The curl of my lips,

I'm a woman,

Phenomenally.

Phenomenal woman,

That's me."

Maya Angelou

NOTES:

ABOUT THE AUTHOR

Dr. Jacqueline Eubany is a board certified cardiologist and electrophysiologist, who is currently practicing medicine in Orange County, California.

Jacqueline was born in Lagos, Nigeria and attended the University of California Riverside for her undergraduate degree then Boston University for medical school. She joined the United States Navy after medical school and completed her internal medicine residencies at Naval Medical Center San Diego, Cardiovascular Disease fellowship at National Naval Medical Center Bethesda, and electrophysiology fellowship at the George Washington university in Washington DC.

While working as a physician in the US Navy, her clinic was responsible for the healthcare of Active Duty Military, including wounded war veterans returning from Iraq and Afghanistan, and members of congress. She served in the United States Navy for twelve years. She was inducted as a fellow in the prestigious American College of Cardiology, and in the Heart Rhythm Society. She is an active member in other distinguished societies, and has served on several advisory boards related to heart disease. She has been invited to be the guest speaker for several heart health events because she has a major interest in women's heart health.

Dr. Eubany has visited over 50 countries, and enjoys scuba diving, horseback riding, biking and reading about world history.

REFERENCES:

1. Kochanek KD, Xu JQ, Murphy SL, Miniño AM, Kung HC. Deaths: final data for 2009 [PDF-2M]. National vital statistics reports. 2011;60(3).
2. U.S. Department of Health and Human Services, Office on Women's Health. Heart Disease: Frequently Asked Questions. 2009. [cited 2013 July 19, 2013]; Available from: http://www.womenshealth.gov/publications/ourp ublications/fact-sheet/heart-disease.pdf [PDF-1.7M].
3. Mosca L, Mochari-Greenberger H, Dolor RJ, Newby LK, Robb KJ. Twelve-year follow-up of American women's awareness of cardiovascular disease risk and barriers to heart health. Circulation: Cardiovascular Quality Outcomes. 2010;3:120-7.
4. National Heart, Lung and Blood Institute. What Are the Signs and Symptoms of Heart Disease? [cited 2013 July 19, 2013]; Available from: www.nhlbi.nih.gov/health/health-topics/hdw/signs.html.
5. Heron M. Deaths: Leading causes for 2008 [PDF-2.7M]. National vital statistics reports. 2012;60(6).
6. Roger VL, Go AS, Lloyd-Jones DM, Benjamin EJ, Berry JD, Borden WB, et al. Heart disease and stroke statistics— 2012 update: a report from the American Heart Association. Circulation. 2012;125(1): e2–220.
7. CDC. Million Hearts: strategies to reduce the prevalence of leading cardiovascular disease risk

factors. United States, 2011. MMWR 2011;60(36):1248–51.

8. National Heart, Lung and Blood Institute. What Are the Signs and Symptoms of Heart Disease? [cited 2013 July 19, 2013]; Available from: www.nhlbi.nih.gov/health/health-topics/hdw/signs.html.

9. Centers for Disease Control and Prevention. Smoking-Attributable Mortality, Years of Potential Life Lost, and Productivity Losses — United States, 2000–2004. Morbidity and Mortality Weekly Report. November 14, 2008; 57(45):1226–28.

10. Centers for Disease Control and Prevention. National Center for Chronic Disease Prevention and Health Promotion. Tobacco Information and Prevention Source (TIPS). Tobacco Use in the United States. January 27, 2004.

11. Centers for Disease Control and Prevention. Cigarette Smoking Attributable Morbidity — U.S., 2000. Morbidity and Mortality Weekly Report. 2003 Sept; 52(35): 842-844.

12. U.S Department of Health and Human Services. Health Consequences of Smoking: A Report of the Surgeon General, 2004.

13. Centers for Disease Control and Prevention. Annual Smoking-Attributable Mortality, Years of Potential Life Lost, and Economic Costs — United States, 1995–1999. Morbidity and Mortality Weekly Report. April 12, 2002; 51(14):300-3.

14. U.S. Department of Health and Human Services. Women and Smoking: A Report of the Surgeon General, 2001.
15. Centers for Disease Control and Prevention. National Center for Health Statistics. National Vital Statistics Reports. Births: Final Data for 2005. December 5, 2007; (56)5.
16. Centers for Disease Control and Prevention. State Estimates of Neonatal Health-Care Costs Associated with Maternal Smoking — United States, 1996. Morbidity and Mortality Weekly Report. October 8, 2004; 53(39):915-917.
17. Centers for Disease Control and Prevention. National Center for Health Statistics. National Health Interview Survey, 2009. Analysis by the American Lung Association, Research and Program Services Division using SPSS and SUDAAN software
18. Ibid.
19. Ibid.
20. Centers for Disease Control and Prevention. Youth Risk Behavior Surveillance — United States, 2009. Morbidity and Mortality Weekly Report. June 4, 2010; 59(SS-05).
21. Centers for Disease Control and Prevention. Office on Smoking and Health. National Youth Tobacco Survey, 2009. Analysis by the American Lung Association, Research and Program Services Division using SPSS software.
22. U.S. Federal Trade Commission. Cigarette Report for 2006. August 2009. Accessed on September 24, 2009.

23. U.S. Department of Health and Human Services. Preventing Tobacco Use among Young People: A Report of the Surgeon General, 1994. U.S. Department of Health and Human Services. The. Atlanta: U.S. Department of Health and Human Services, Centers for Disease Control and Prevention, National Center for Chronic Disease Prevention and Health Promotion, Office on Smoking and Health, 2014 [accessed 2014 October 29].

24. Fiore MC, Jaén CR, Baker TB, Bailey WC, Benowitz NL, Curry SJ, Dorfman SF, Froelicher ES, Goldstein MG, Froelicher ES, Healton CG, et al. Treating Tobacco Use and Dependence: 2008 Update—Clinical Practice Guidelines. Rockville (MD): U.S. Department of Health and Human Services, Public Health Service, Agency for Healthcare Research and Quality, 2008 [accessed 2014 October 29].

25. U.S. Department of Health and Human Services. How Tobacco Smoke Causes Disease: The Biology and Behavioral Basis for Smoking-Attributable Disease: A Report of the Surgeon General. Atlanta: U.S. Department of Health and Human Services, Centers for Disease Control and Prevention, National Center for Chronic Disease Prevention and Health Promotion, Office on Smoking and Health, 2010 [accessed 2014 October 29].

26. U.S. Department of Health and Human Services. Reducing Tobacco Use: A Report of the Surgeon General. Atlanta: U.S. Department of Health and Human Services, Centers for Disease Control and Human Services, Centers for Disease Control and

Prevention, National Center for Chronic Disease
Prevention and Health Promotion, Office on
Smoking and Health, 2000 [accessed 2014 October
29].

27. National Institute on Drug Abuse. Research Report
Series: Tobacco Addiction. Bethesda (MD):
National Institutes of Health, National Institute on
Drug Abuse, 2009 [accessed 2014 October 29].

28. American Society of Addiction Medicine. Public
Policy Statement on Nicotine Dependence and
Tobacco. Chevy Chase (MD): American Society of
Addiction Medicine, 2010 [accessed 2014 October
29].

29. National Toxicology Program. Report on
Carcinogens, Twelfth Edition. Research Triangle
Park (NC): U.S. Department of Health and Human
Sciences, National Institute of Environmental
Health Sciences, National Toxicology Program,
2011 [accessed 2014 October 29].

30. U.S. Department of Health and Human Services.
The Health Consequences of Smoking: A Report of
the Surgeon General. Atlanta: U.S. Department of
Health and Human Services, Centers for Disease
Control and Prevention, National Center for
Chronic Disease Prevention and Health Promotion,
Office on Smoking and Health, 2004 [accessed
2014 October 29].

31. U.S. Department of Health and Human Services.
The Health Benefits of Smoking Cessation: A
Report of the Surgeon General. Atlanta: U.S.
Department of Health and Human Services, Centers

for Disease Control and Prevention, Center for Chronic Disease Prevention and Health Promotion, Office on Smoking and Health, 1990 [accessed 2014 October 29].

32. Centers for Disease Control and Prevention. Quitting Smoking Among Adults—United States, 2001–2010. Morbidity and Mortality Weekly Report 2011;60(44):1513–19 [accessed 2014 October 29].

33. Centers for Disease Control and Prevention. Youth Risk Behavior Surveillance—United States, 2013. Morbidity and Mortality Weekly Report [serial online] 2014;63(SS–4):1–168 [accessed 2014 October 29].

34. Centers for Disease Control and Prevention. Community Guide Community Preventive Services: Reducing Tobacco Use and Secondhand Smoke Exposure [page last updated 2014 Jan 30; accessed 2014 October 29].

35. U.S. Food and Drug Administration The FDA Approves Novel Medication for Smoking Cessation. FDA Consumer, 2006 [cited 2014 October 29].

36. Mowery PD, Brick PD, Farrelly MC. Legacy First Look Report 3. Pathways to Established Smoking: Results from the 1999 National Youth Tobacco Survey. Washington DC: American Legacy Foundation. October 2000.

37. California Environmental Protection Agency. Proposed Identification of Environmental Tobacco Smoke as a Toxic Air Contaminant: Executive Summary. June 24, 2005.

38. California Environmental Protection Agency. Proposed Identification of Environmental Tobacco Smoke as a Toxic Air Contaminant. June 2005.

39. Shopland DR, Gerlach KK, Burns DM, Hartman AM, Gibson JT. State-Specific Trends in Smoke-free Workplace Policy Coverage: The Current Population Tobacco Use Supplement, 1993 to 1999. Journal of Occupational and Environmental Medicine. August, 2001; 43(8):680-6.

40. Centers for Disease Control and Prevention. National Center for Health Statistics. National Health Interview Survey, 2009. Analysis by the American Lung Association, Research and Program Services Division using SPSS and SUDAAN software.

41. National Institute of Drug Abuse. Research Report on Nicotine: Addiction, August 2001.

42. Fiore MC, Jaen CR, Baker TB, et al. Treating Tobacco Use and Dependence: 2008 Update. Clinical Practice Guideline. Rockville, MD: U.S. Department of Health and Human Services. Public Health Service. May 2008.

43. U.S. Department of Health and Human Services. Reducing Tobacco Use: A Report of the Surgeon General 2000.

44. U.S. Department of Health and Human Services, U.S. Department of Agriculture (2010). *Dietary Guidelines for Americans, 2010*, 7th ed. Washington, DC: US.
http://www.healthierus.gov/dietaryguideline

45. Johnson RK, et al. (2009). Dietary sugars intake and cardiovascular health: A scientific statement from the American Heart Association. *Circulation*, 120(11):1011-1020
46. www.dashdiet.org
47. www.mayoclinic.org
48. Halton TL, Willett WC, Liu S, et. Al. *Low-carbohydrate diet score and risk of coronary heart disease in women*. N Engl J Med.2006;355:1991-2002
49. Halton TL, Liu S, Manson JE, Hu FB. *Low-carbohydrate-diet score and risk of type 2 diabetes in women*. Am J Clin Nutr.2008;87:339-46
50. Patel, S.R. and F.B. Hu. *Short sleep duration and weight gain: a systematic review*. Obesity (Silver Spring), 2008.16(3):643-53
51. Patel, S.R., et al. Association between reduced sleep and weight gain in women. Am J Epidemiol,2006.164(10):947-54
52. Berrington de Gonzalez, A., et al., *Body-mass-index and mortality among 1.46 million white adults*. N Engl J Med,2010.363(23):2211-9
53. Willett W, Nutritional epidemiology. 1998.New York: oxford University Press.
54. Clinical Guidelines on the Identification, Evaluation, and Treatment of Overweight and Obesity in Adults-The Evidence Report. National Institutes of health. Obes Res,1998.6Suppl 2:51s-209s
55. Zhang, X., et al., Abdominal obesity and the risk of all-cause, cardiovascular, and cancer mortality:

sixteen years of follow-up in US women. Circulation,2008.117(13):1658

56. Pemu,PI,Offili,E. Hypertension in women. J Clin Hypertension 2008;10406

57. Aronow et al., ACCF/AHA 2011 expert consensus document on hypertension in the elderly: a report of the ACC Foundation Task Force on Clinical Expert Consensus Document Developed in collaboration with AAN, AGS, ASPC, ASH, ASN; ABC, and ESH. Journal of the American Society of Hypertension:5(4):259-352

58. High cholesterolFedder DO, Koro CE, L'italien GJ. New National Cholesterol Education Program III for primary prevention lipid-lowering drug therapy: projected impact on the size, sex and age distribution of the treatment-eligible population. CIRC 2002;105;152

59. Grundy SM, Cleeman JI, Merz CN. Et al. Implications of recent clinical trials for the National Cholesterol Education Program Adult Treatment Panel III guidelines. Circ 2004:110:227

60. www.health.harvard.edu

61. www.aha.org

62. www.emedcinehealth.com

63. "Diabetes Fact Sheet N 312. WHO. October 2013. Retrieved 25 March 2014.

64. "Update 2014". IDF. International Diabetes Federation. Retrieved 29 November 2014.

65. Williams textbook endocrinology (12th ed.). Philadelphia: Elsevier/Saunders.

66. Shi, Yuankai; et al. "The global implication of diabetes and cancer". The Lance 383 (9933): 1947-8

67. "The top 10 causes of death fact sheet N 310. WHO. Oct 2013

68. "National Diabetes Clearinghouse: National Diabetes Statistics 2011

69. Mosca, Lori et al. Hormone Replacement Therapy and Cardiovascular Disease: A statement for healthcare professionals from the American Heart Association. Circulation 2001; 104:499-503

70. Hormone therapy and heart disease. Committee Opinion No. 565. American College of Obstetrician and Gynecologists. Obstet Gynecol 2013; 121:1407-10

71. Barrett-Connor E. Hormones and heart disease in women: the timing hypothesis. Am J Epidemiol 2007; 166:506-10

72. Manson JE, Bassuk SS. Invited commentary: hormone therapy and risk of coronary heart disease why renew the focus on the early years of menopause? Am J Epidemiol 2007; 166:511-7

73. Barrett-Connor E, Bush TL. Estrogen and coronary heart disease in women. JAMA 1991; 265:1861-7. [PubMed] ⇐

74. Grady D, Rubin SM, Petitti DB, Fox CS, Black D, Ettinger B, et al. Hormone therapy to prevent disease and prolong life in postmenopausal women. Ann Intern Med 1992; 117:1016-37. [PubMed] ⇐

75. Barrett-Connor E, Grady D. Hormone replacement therapy, heart disease, and other considerations. Annu Rev Public Health 1998; 19:55–72. [PubMed] ⇐

76. Rossouw JE, Anderson GL, Prentice RL, LaCroix AZ, Kooperberg C, Stefanick ML, et al. Risks and benefits of estrogen plus progestin in healthy postmenopausal women: principal results From the Women's Health Initiative randomized controlled trial. Writing Group for the Women's Health Initiative Investigators. JAMA 2002; 288:321–33. [PubMed] [Full Text] ⇐

77. Hulley S, Grady D, Bush T, Furberg C, Herrington D, Riggs B, et al. Randomized trial of estrogen plus progestin for secondary prevention of coronary heart disease in postmenopausal women. Heart and Estrogen/progestin Replacement Study (HERS) Research Group. JAMA 1998; 280:605–13. [PubMed] [Full Text] ⇐

78. Grady D, Herrington D, Bittner V, Blumenthal R, Davidson M, Hlatky M, et al. Cardiovascular disease outcomes during 6.8 years of hormone therapy: Heart and Estrogen/progestin Replacement Study follow-up (HERS II). HERS Research Group [published erratum appears in JAMA 2002; 288:1064]. JAMA 2002; 288:49–57. [PubMed] [Full Text] ⇐

79. Barrett-Connor E. Hormones and heart disease in women: the timing hypothesis. Am J Epidemiology 2007; 166:506–10. [PubMed] ⇐

80. Manson JE, Bask SS. Invited commentary: hormone therapy and risk of coronary heart disease why renew the focus on the early years of menopause? Am J Epidemiol 2007; 166:511–7. [PubMed] [Full Text] ⇐

81. Hsia J, Langer RD, Manson JE, Kuller L, Johnson KC, Hendrix SL, et al. Conjugated equine estrogens and coronary heart disease: the Women's Health Initiative. Women's Health Initiative Investigators [published erratum appears in Arch Intern Med 2006; 166:759]. Arch Intern Med 2006; 166:357–65. [PubMed] [Full Text] ⇐

82. Simon JA, Hsia J, Cauley JA, Richards C, Harris F, Fong J, et al. Postmenopausal hormone therapy and risk of stroke: The Heart and Estrogen-progestin Replacement Study (HERS). Circulation 2001; 103:638–42. [PubMed] [Full Text] ⇐

83. Grodstein F, Manson JE, Colditz GA, Willett WC, Speizer FE, Stampfer MJ. A prospective, observational study of postmenopausal hormone therapy and primary prevention of cardiovascular disease. Ann Intern Med 2000; 133:933–41. [PubMed] ⇐

84. Manson JE, Hsia J, Johnson KC, Rossouw JE, Assaf AR, Lasser NL, et al. Estrogen plus progestin and the risk of coronary heart disease. Women's Health

Initiative Investigators. N Engl J Med 2003; 349:523–34. [PubMed] [Full Text] ⇐

85. Rossouw JE, Prentice RL, Manson JE, Wu L, Barad D, Barnabei VM, et al. Postmenopausal hormone therapy and risk of cardiovascular disease by age and years since menopause [published erratum appears in JAMA 2008; 299:1426]. JAMA 2007; 297:1465–77. [PubMed] [Full Text] ⇐

86. Manson JE, Allison MA, Rossouw JE, Carr JJ, Langer RD, Hia J, et al. Estrogen therapy and coronary-artery calcification. WHI and WHI-CACS Investigators. N Engl J Med 2007; 356:2591–602. [PubMed] [Full Text] ⇐

87. Allison MA, Manson JE, Langer RD, Carr JJ, Rossouw JE, Pettinger MB, et al. Oophorectomy, hormone therapy, and subclinical coronary artery disease in women with hysterectomy: the Women's Health Initiative coronary artery calcium study. Women's Health Initiative and Women's Health Initiative Coronary Artery Calcium Study Investigators. Menopause 2008; 15:639–47. [PubMed] [Full Text] ⇐

88. Bernstein P, Pohost G. Progesterone, progestin's, and the heart. Rev Cardiovasc Med 2010; 11:228–36. [PubMed] ⇐

89. Rosano GM, Webb CM, Chierchia S, Morgani GL, Gabraele M, Sarrel PM, et al. Natural progesterone, but not medroxyprogesterone acetate, enhances the beneficial effect of estrogen on exercise-

induced myocardial ischemia in postmenopausal women. J Am Coll Cardiol 2000;36: 2154–9. [PubMed] [Full Text] ⇐

90. Rylance PB, Brincat M, Lafferty K, De Trafford JC, Brincat S, Parsons V, et al. Natural progesterone and antihypertensive action. Br Med J (Clin Res Ed) 1985; 290:13–4. [PubMed] [Full Text] ⇐

91. Lee DY, Kim JY, Kim JH, Choi DS, Kim DK, Koh KK, et al. Effects of hormone therapy on ambulatory blood pressure in postmenopausal Korean women. Climacteric 2011; 14:92–9. [PubMed] [Full Text] ⇐

92. Cook N, Min Lee I, Buring J. Women's Health Study: A randomized controlled trial. JAMA 2005; 294:56-65

93. Vivekananthan DP, et al. Use of antioxidant vitamins for the prevention of cardiovascular disease: meta-analyses of randomized trials 2003. Lancet 2003 June 14; 361:2017-23

94. Lee IM, Cook NR, Gaziano JM, et al. Vitamin E in the primary prevention of cardiovascular disease and cancer: the Women's Health Study: A randomized controlled trial. JAMA. 2005; 294:56-65

95. Lonn E, Bosch J, Yusuf S, et al. Effects of long-term vitamin E supplementation on cardiovascular events and cancer a randomized controlled trial. JAMA. 2005; 293:1338-47

96. McSweeney J, et al. Women's Early Warning Symptoms of Acute Myocardial Infarction. Circulation 2003; 108:2619-23